YOGA
shakti

YOGA
shakti

AWAKEN YOUR OWN POWER

SHAILAJA MENON

With a Foreword by **Shashi Tharoor**

NIYOGI
BOOKS

Published by
NIYOGI BOOKS
Block D, Building No. 77,
Okhla Industrial Area, Phase-I,
New Delhi-110 020, INDIA
Tel: 91-11-26816301, 26818960
Email: niyogibooks@gmail.com
Website: www.niyogibooksindia.com

Editor: Jyotika Mansata
Design: Shashi Bhushan Prasad

ISBN: 978-93-86906-44-1
Publication: 2018

Printed at: Niyogi Offset Pvt. Ltd., New Delhi, India

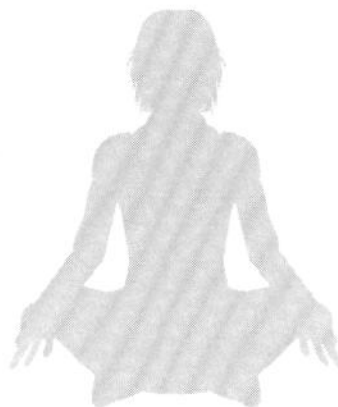

To my father, the late Dr V. Jayakumaran, who set the bar for me to live a larger life by his own life's work, through which he touched countless lives.

To my mother, Sushila Jayakumaran, for the experience of unconditional love.

To my husband, Prem, and my sons, Vyshnav and Krishan, for bringing stability and joy into my life.

To Manoj Kaimal, My Teacher, Founder, Manasa Yoga, for inspiring me to evolve towards expressing my highest potential.

To the Gurus, for the great wisdom and teachings that have been passed on through the passage of time.

To Shakti, the primordial pulsating cosmic energy of consciousness

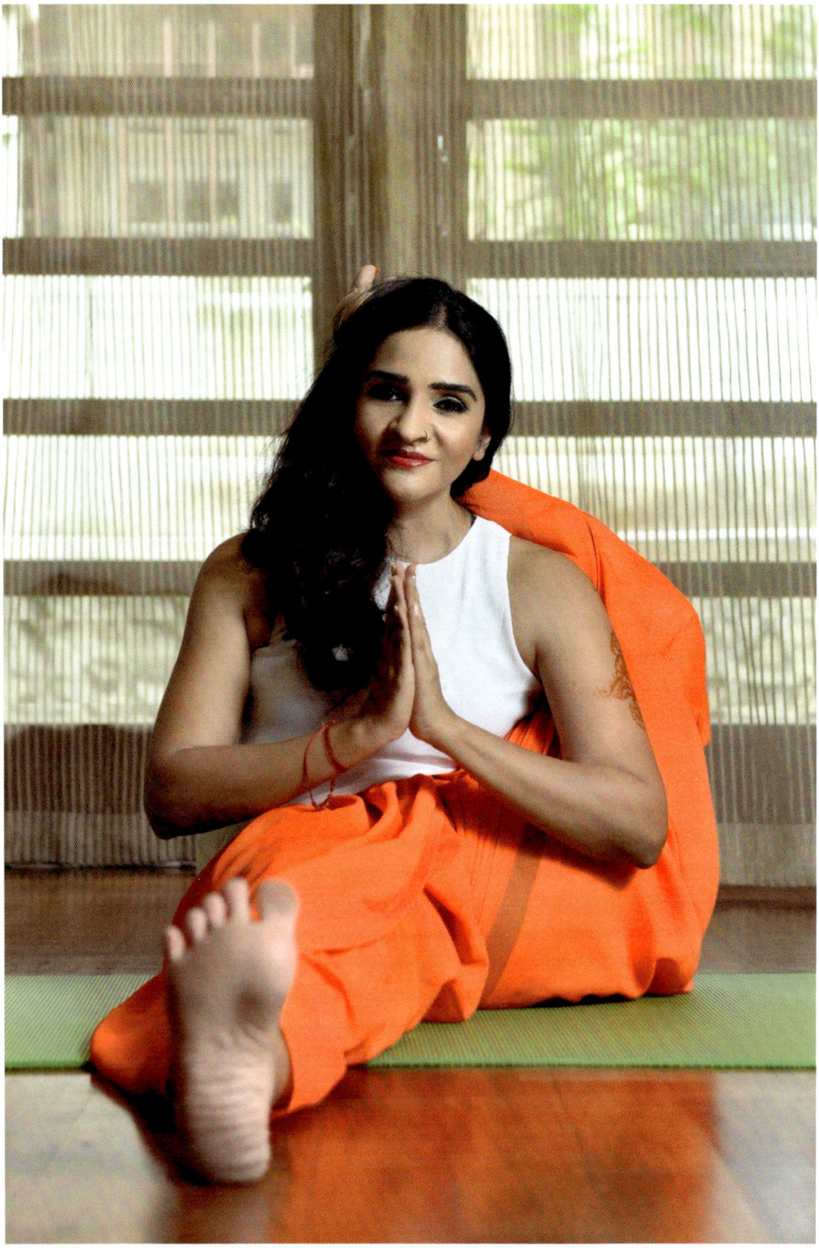

Eka Pada Sirsasana or Foot Behind the Head Pose

Contents

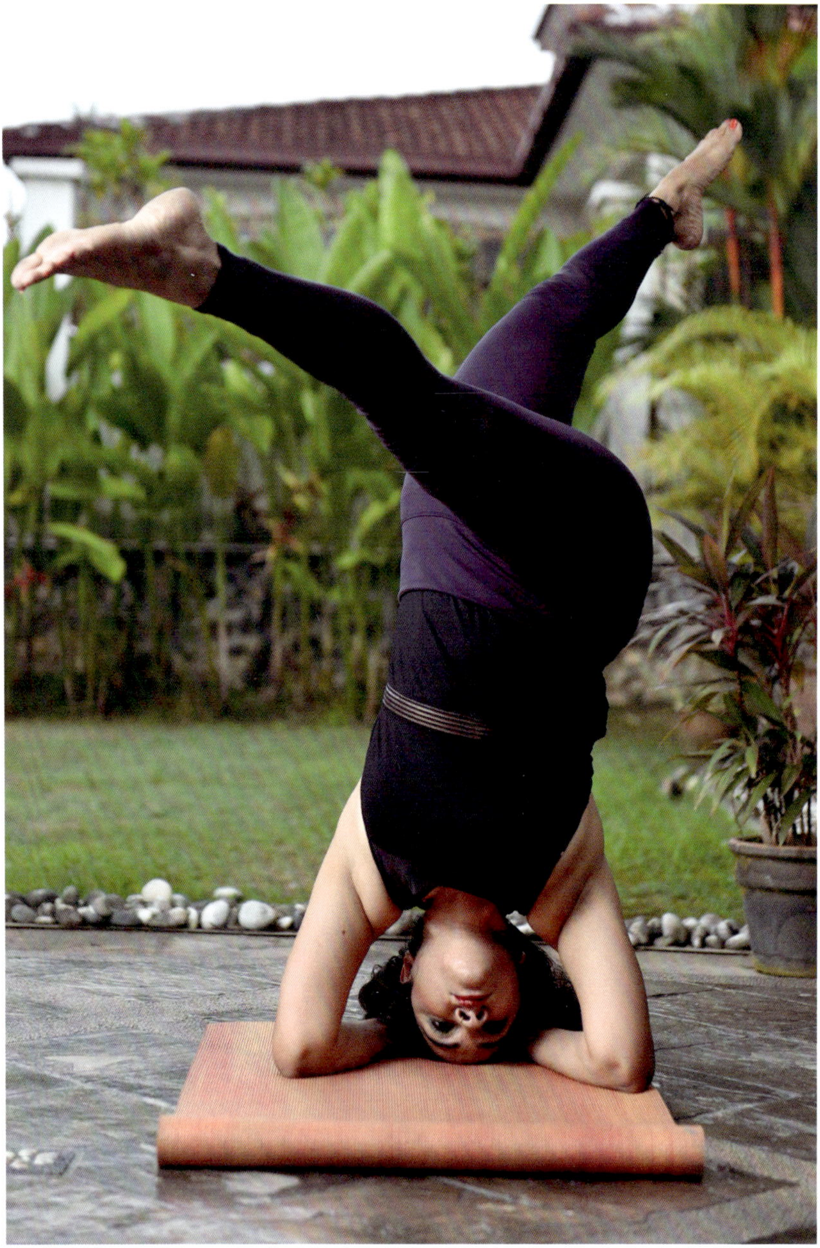

Parivrttaikapada Sirsasana or Revolved Split-Legged Headstand

Acknowledgements

This list is surely incomplete as there are so many people who have shaped my life over the years, but I am confining this to those who have shaped this book and my yogic path over the years.

My deepest gratitude to:

Dr Shashi Tharoor, Member of Parliament for Thiruvananthapuram and author, who took the time out from his extremely busy schedule, to write a Foreword in support of my book and the cause of yoga.

Kamlesh Barwal, International Director, Sri Sri Yoga; Shirley Telles, Director, Patanjali Research Foundation; Tunku Halim, Malaysian novelist, short-story and non-fiction writer and lawyer, for generously taking the time to read and share their views on my book in their own inimitable styles.

Dr Kausthub Desikachar, for his faith in the book. He unreservedly shared his publishing expertise and guided me to gain the right support for the book.

Mataji Divyananda, who first inspired me on the path of yoga 18 years ago, by embodying the love, patience, peace and wisdom I sought.

Mini Padmam, who championed the book from its very first page, reading chapter after chapter, encouraging me every step of the way as I was writing it

Sharad Nair, for the vital role he has played in ensuring the success of my book.

Janaki Surendranath, who was one of the first people to encourage me to write the book, even going as far as to compile and send me a list of publishers, one of which was Niyogi Books.

Vinay Kumar, who sensed my dedication to the yoga practice and supported me through his prolific writings on yoga in our Facebook group, 'Live n Joy'.

My students at 'Mat and Beyond Yoga Studio' and everywhere else, who resonate with my words and find value in my teachings. You inspire me to continue my work with your commitment to the practice and the beautiful blossoming of your lives.

Lakshmi Narayanan in Singapore, who patiently shared her vast experience in the realm of publishing with me.

My friends at the Manasa yoga student community, some of whom I have practiced alongside for many years now.

My family: my mother-in-law, Sarojini, who has wholeheartedly supported me over the years; my siblings and their spouses, Narayanan and Meera, Radhika and Manoj; my uncle M.K. Vijayshanker; my aunts, Chandrika and Indira.

My friends, Karti and Senthil, who are my family back home in Coimbatore; my good friends here in Malaysia, Viji, Anju, Sushmita, Liza ... the list is incomplete and I thank you all for your support over the years.

My publishers, Niyogi Books, for their faith in the book.

Foreword

Yoga is perhaps one of the most powerful traditions known to us. Across time and culture, the teachings of yogic philosophy have brought tremendous meditative and spiritual solace to its practitioners. Whether in helping deepen our devotion to God or in enriching our service to others, yoga paves a path towards self-realization and contentment that has uplifted individuals and strengthened societies for centuries.

Yet, the discipline also remains poorly understood. Although yoga has seen unprecedented diffusion into popular culture, awareness of its spiritual benefits is often diluted through its contemporary commercialization and politicization. The costs of such distortion are high: as we witness societies fracture across differences and individuals fall victim to new stresses, the need to understand and practice yoga in its truest form is felt acutely. We must remember that the fruits of yoga are borne not only from its physical performance, but in the changes that occur beneath the surface to instil habits of compassion and feelings of peace.

In this context, *Yoga Shakti* serves as a reminder that is as refreshing as it is vital. By drawing from her own journey, Shailaja reinvigorates the discipline with candour, discipline, and a genuine desire to share the benefits she has herself felt. She communicates the lessons of the Patanjali Sutras to emphasize the spiritual purpose of yoga, in a manner that remains loyal to the intentions of its scholars while being accessible to today's audiences.

In doing so, Shailaja allows readers to navigate their own feelings of agitation, depression, and restlessness, while helping them find direction through the yogic teachings of asana and *atha*. By exploring the fundamental tenets of yoga, addressing the questions of laymen, and suggesting daily exercises, *Yoga Shakti* revives the philosophical roots of yoga and provides a comprehensive guide that enlightens both the curious and the informed. I thoroughly recommend it to all who seek self-realization through the power of yoga.

Dr Shashi Tharoor

Preface

Yoga is a vast subject with diverse philosophies coursing through it. In our system, Manasa yoga, we focus primarily on the dualistic *Yoga Sutras* of Patanjali, the non-dualistic Advaita Vedanta of Adi Shankaracharya, and the non-dualistic doctrines of Kashmir Shaivism. Etched out in the architecture of these great edifices of amazing insights are beautiful maps which reveal the entire topography of consciousness. The two poles which we generally find in these maps would be of samsara (entanglement and suffering) on one end, and samadhi (wisdom and liberation) on the other. Samsara refers to the repeated cycles of life, a place of entanglement and suffering, and samadhi refers to a series of insightful absorptions which disentangles us and liberates us from this endless cycle of suffering.

Generally, the context of liberation points to a release from the mundane world and an absorption into the supramundane. However, this binary view of dystopic immanence and utopic transcendence is not the direction of our system of yoga. What we really want is for students to understand the maps of yoga teachings, which will then reveal the terrains of their own consciousness, and help them realize where they currently operate from.

Here, the schematic framing of thought patterns and capacities into the unwholesome (*ashuba vasanas*) and wholesome (*shuba vasanas*) help us to sharpen our capacity of discernment. With this sharpened sword of intellect (*viveka*), we can sever the tentacles of self-defeating thought patterns (*samskaras*) which were only raised in ignorance (*avidya*), and subsequently allow for the blossoming of wholesome patterns which serve in helping us reach our highest potential.

So instead of focusing on being released from the different recurring challenges of life (samsara), the yoga practitioner finds himself/ herself learning from each cycle, getting enriched in the process, and being able to conduct themselves more skillfully. Not only do they not suffer, but they are able to deeply relish the gift of embodied life. And in the whole process, the student's awareness and perception expands to not only sense the body and mind, but also the presence of a hierarchically organized order of underlying energy and intelligence, much like the famous ontological concepts of the explicate order and the implicate order of the great theoretical physicist David Bohm.

As we walk this path, in what was previously the immanent, we experience the transcendent. Instead of liberation, we celebrate our individuality. We reclaim our true power. This is the direction which Shailaja will take you through this book.

Shailaja first walked into my class around 15 years ago. She had already been practicing yoga for several years before coming to our studio. Perhaps the focus of the Manasa yoga system, in the simultaneous threading of each asana with precise biomechanical considerations along with transformational philosophical contemplations, is what intrigued and inspired her, and kept her coming regularly to my classes. In this period I saw her transform, from a student keen on the shape aspects of asana to a very contemplative practitioner, probing deep into both physique and psyche to experientially realize the various coalesced states of mind and body, action and reflection, *Siva* and Sakti, *Jiva* and Atma, in short—consciousness and energy. Her explorations, along with the different insights she received while going through the crucible of life is evident in her writing. These insights will help anyone going through the different challenges that life offers.

I end my note with this share of a line of the great Tantric mystic Kshemaraja, who sang in ecstasy—'*dharanitahsadantamsivaya, everything in this universe, from the mundane to the supra mundane, from the waste on the pavement to the deity in the sanctum sanctorum, are all refractions of the ONE great light.*'

May we too be able to sing the same, rejoicing in our inherent oneness while respecting the apparent differences between us.

It is with great pride that I write this Preface for her book. I wish Shailaja and all the readers of this book the very best.

Manoj Kaimal
Founder, Manasa Yoga

Disclaimer

The yoga asanas written about and demonstrated in this book are of an intermediate level to embody certain qualities of the heart. They should only be practiced under the guidance of an experienced teacher.

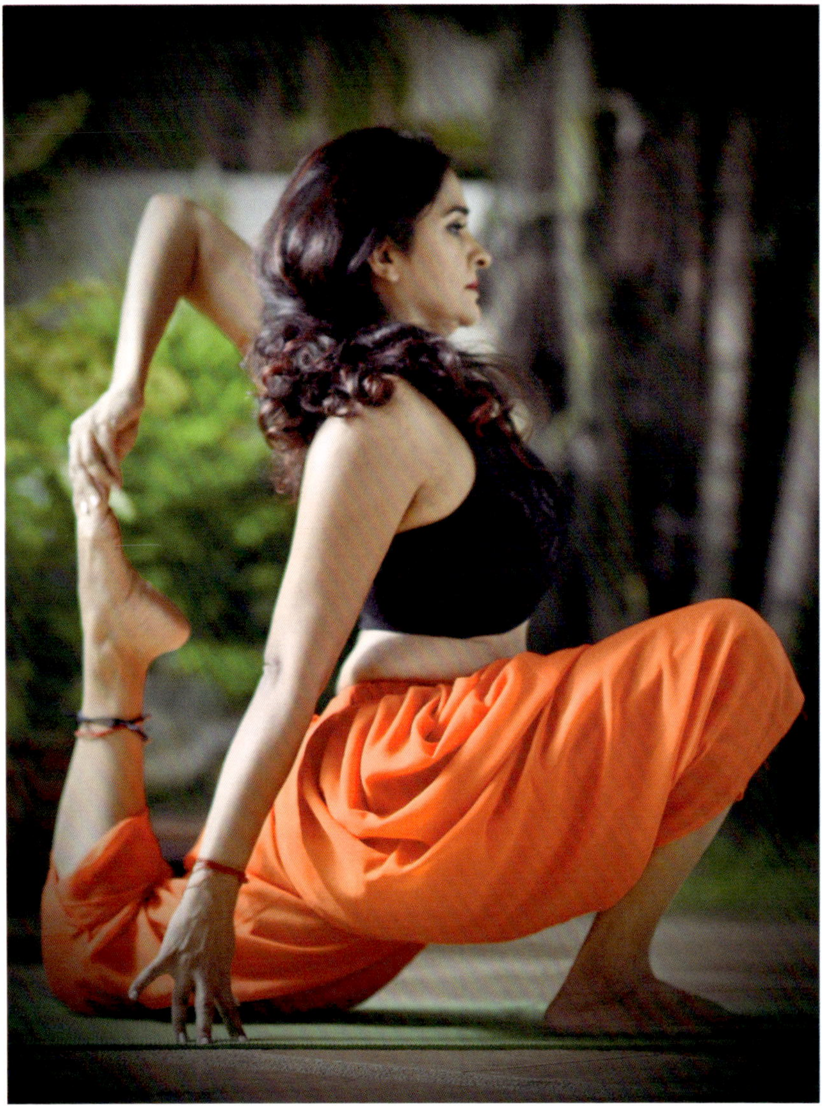

Artistic Pose: *Ekapada Raja Kapotasana* or One-legged King Pigeon Pose

Aham Brahmasmi: I Am That

The core of my being is the ultimate reality, the root and ground of the universe, the source of all that exists.

Most of us, even as adults, give our power away. It is an unconscious giving away, insidiously ingrained in us from as far back as we can remember. From childhood we are trained to look outwards, seek answers outside of ourselves—from parents, teachers, elders, bosses, friends, gurus, just about everybody except ourselves! From childhood, our Indian culture discourages us to question the status quo. In fact, it is considered rude and even disrespectful to question what we are told to do or follow. We are trained to believe that other people, by virtue of their position, relationship status or age, know better. We are conditioned to live our lives and base our decisions on other people's opinions, and society's expectations.

The emphasis in life is mostly on the outside world; excel in school, get admission into a good university (preferably Ivy League), party with friends, engage in relationships, and get great jobs. Expectations are set young, and children usually just go with the flow. A lot of our life is already predetermined, even before we are born, by our race, our nationality, our religion (Hindu, Christian, Buddhist, Muslim, Jain) our language, our food (eat beef/pork, don't eat beef/pork, halal, vegetarian, no garlic and onions please!), the way we dress (sari, salwar kurta, spaghetti straps or burkha), our expected manner of behaviour, societal/parental/familial expectations of what we should study (medicine, engineering, accountancy), when we should get married, who we should marry, and even how many times we can get married!

Quo Vadis: Whither Goest Thou?

When we are disconnected from ourselves, our minds and our lives lack clarity and purpose. We are constantly searching for 'meaning in life', and we experience it in our minds as states of restlessness and agitation. We are not sure of what our lives are about. The 'path' eludes us and we are left with more questions than answers. It may appear on the surface that our lives are perfect as we get on with the tasks of working, socializing, raising a family etc., yet deep inside us a sense of emptiness gnaws, surfacing at the most inopportune times with disquieting regularity. To counter that we may turn to food, which results in over eating, to alcohol and cigarettes, which leads to fatal addictions, or wild outbursts of anger or sadness that destabilize our minds and our lives. We may experience deep feelings of jealousy and envy as we see others blossom in their chosen paths, socialize irresponsibly, and feel a deep restlessness that manifests as an inability to stick with a job or relationship. Over a period of time these patterns only takes us deeper into the quagmire. We keep looking outward through relationships and jobs, but the world is not designed to cater to us. Relationships end and divorce statistics are at an all-time high. In this current economic climate, with restructuring and cost cutting being the order of the day, people are losing jobs and being displaced. Even our children leave home and move on at some point. Everything in our outer worlds is subject to the relentless principle of flux.

When we feel lost and unsure of what our lives are about, or some terrible tragedy befalls us and we are unable to summon the strength to carry on, then the wisdom of the spiritual teachings passed down through the ages offers us direction. We consciously seek out teachers or attend religious discourses, seeking meaning and solace. Many a time it is the beacon of light that guides us out of the woods, so to speak. The teachings offer hope, inspiration, clarity and motivation to get out of bed and stay on the path, even when feelings like anger, anxiety and depression threaten to drag us down and keep us there. At a deeper level we may even require it, like a salve for the mind, as at that point in our lives we may be past knowing what is good for us, what the next best thing to do is, and where we go from that point. So we place our trust and judgment in the hands of someone we look up to, someone we hold with the highest trust—our teacher.

At the outset let me tell you that I have the greatest regard for teachers (being a teacher myself) and gurus. These relationships and connections are sacred. They open our minds from our limited egocentric perspective of 'I, Me, Myself', and from the conditioned ideas and notions that we hold about how life should be or people should behave. True teachers uplift us from our 'smallness' and inspire us to reach our highest potential. From a teacher we ostensibly gain knowledge, yet, through their eyes, we are blessed with glimpses of the grand vision of our greater expanded selves.

So what is the problem with that? The problem is that we get stuck. The teachings are meant to release us, to serve in the evolution and unfolding of our greater selves. Yet, if we are not conscious and do not connect to the essence of the teachings, it becomes more about deifying the teacher. We succumb to the all-too-human tendency to attach ourselves to someone or something. And whenever we get stuck, we do not grow. In time, we become almost compulsively dependent, without ever getting on the path to connecting with our inner selves.

When we operate on blind faith, we hand over the reins of our thought process to someone else. Our innate intelligence and ability to think and rationalize goes into deep freeze. When we always look to someone else for answers, we miss the opportunity to connect to our inner guidance system. In fact, many of us are not even aware that we have one! Some people may even find the very idea blasphemous—that we should listen to our inner voice as opposed to a parent, teacher, priest, preacher or society.

We can't hope to fulfill our tryst with destiny by leading someone else's life.

We give our power away when we let other people set the rules, when we allow them to dictate our choices based on their conditioning and their interpretation of situations, events, and scriptures. I have seen the same sutra or verse in the scriptures being interpreted in many different ways in different books by different teachers! By putting people on a pedestal, we open up spaces and opportunities for people to take advantage of our vulnerability and our weakness, even abuse it, which has been demonstrated time and time again across the globe; from the rampant sexual abuse of children in the Catholic Church, to the many instances of abuse in our ashrams, to cults that form suicide pacts! Absolute power has an unequivocally corrupting effect, and the case is no different in the field of religion or spirituality.

All this stems from a general lack of awareness of our own

capacity to connect to the infinite intelligence within us, to consciously cultivate that connection, to live in alignment with it and express ourselves from that space.

> *Always remember, truth cannot be said, it can be shown. It is a finger pointing to the moon. All words are just fingers pointing to the moon, but don't accept the fingers as the moon. The moment you start clinging to the finger—that's when doctrines, cults, dogmas, creeds are born—then you have missed the whole point. The fingers were not the point. The point was the moon.*[1]
>
> —Osho

Disconnected Lives

As a result of all this outward looking, as adults we lead disconnected lives. We have a certain inner calling, but because we are not in tune with ourselves, we seldom hear it, much less act on it. We continue to make choices and shape our lives based on archaic conditioning and belief systems we inherit from generations before us. Even today, I have parents tell me how they want (read: insist) their sons or daughters to become doctors because they have to take over their 'family hospital business'! Their intentions are surely good, but it does not take into account the child's own *svadharma,* his inner nature. And they may be unintentionally setting him/her up to a lifetime of struggle to find inner fulfillment.

What is our seed potential? What are we supposed to become? What activities support and nourish our nature? What brings us joy? What activities are effortless and natural for us to engage in? As the clutter in the mind is released, as the waves of agitation and

1 Bhagwan Shree Rajneesh, *The Sword and the Lotus* (Köln, Germany: Rebel Publishing House, 1989).

reactivity settle, we connect to our inner nature and create space for our potential to manifest. As we live and express ourselves authentically from that space, we realize our seed potential and evolve into our highest selves.

Courage—the Defining Factor

And we continue to live like this, either because we are so steeped in unawareness or because we lack the courage to do things differently—to live by our own rules, to write our own script, to walk to the beat of our own drum. Yes, it takes great courage to step outside of our comfort zones, to release every pre-conceived notion of ourselves, to break societal norms and conditioning. In the different areas of our lives—whether as a student who is choosing a path to pursue or in the area of relationships, it takes great courage to speak the truth at the cost of disappointing or hurting the people we love the most; but speak our truth we must if we are to keep our tryst with destiny. Here's one of my all-time favourite quotes to inspire you:

> *I'll make you this promise on your deathbed, in the twilight of your life, it will not be all the risks you took that you will regret the most. Rather, what will fill your heart with the greatest amount of regret and sadness will be all those risks that you did not take, all those opportunities you did not seize and all those fears you did not face. Remember, on the other side of fear lies freedom.*[2]
>
> —Robin Sharma

My Journey

At the end of the day, life is a personal affair. Only we know ourselves, our motivations and intentions, and we have to live

2 Robin Sharma, *Who Will Cry When You Die?* (Mumbai: Jaico Publishing House, 2009).

with the consequences of our choices and our actions. Growing up, I was very unaware of myself; what was it that brought me joy? What inspired me? What motivated me? What values were important to me? What came naturally to me? What did I struggle with? And because of this, I had to make detours in my path.

My brother is a doctor and my sister is an engineer. Since I didn't know what I wanted or where my interests lay, and because I was eager to earn approval in my father's eyes and in the eyes of society, on the advice of well-meaning relatives, I chose to take up chartered accountancy. No surprise, it never worked out. The whole experience scarred me and dented my already vulnerable self-esteem. I was very lost for a long time trying to figure out the clichéd, 'meaning and purpose' in life, and it took me years of soul searching to discover my path. Today I know that I have the least interest in numbers and figures and that it was an area that I should never have ventured into! Yet, I take heart that I learnt early, that all-important lesson of following your heart and doing only what you feel passionate about! Life is too short for anything else! It was a lesson I learnt well.

When Life Comes Crashing Down

It is only when life comes crashing down—we lose a job, we are devastated by the end of a relationship or marriage, we have a bad accident, receive a diagnosis that cripples us or brings us face-to-face with our own mortality—that we delve deeper into everything that we had taken for granted so far. We begin to explore the meaning and mystery of life and relationships, and release the narrow, conditioned and judgmental lens that we viewed life through, in exchange for a broader perspective.

Only in darkness do we realize the value of light, only in ill-health do we truly value a healthy body and mind. Likewise, when we are disconnected from ourselves by giving too much of ourselves to the world through jobs and relationships, we experience severe shocks that jolt us to our very core and turn our worlds upside down. But they have a sacred purpose as they serve as timely reminders of our folly in losing ourselves to the world. They force us to redirect our attention inward, to take responsibility for the state of our lives, and to strengthen our core connection with our inner selves.

The Path of Yoga

Yoga is an inward journey, to connect to the core of ourselves, through the tools of the body, breath and mind. It is a sacred connection that leads us to express our highest possibilities and live authentic and fulfilling lives.

Who is Patanjali? What are the Yoga Sutras?

Patanjali is considered one of the greatest authorities of yoga, and he wrote on three subjects: grammar, medicine and yoga. The *Yoga Sutras* is his culminating work and, through 196 terse aphorisms or sutras—divided into four chapters, he prescribes a path to liberation that ends with man's vision of his true self. The book is a pure exploration of the science of the mind, and one of the earliest and most detailed presentations of the human psyche and consciousness. The book is also very practical, as he provides a path to overcoming the fluctuations of the mind, which are considered major impediments to spiritual development. Though they were written centuries ago, they remain as relevant, fascinating and absorbing, as the nature of man's mind and its fluctuations remain the same.

> *Anyone who tries to sincerely dwell on his writings of the sutras will still feel the pulsating power of transformative spiritual*

teachings throbbing in each of them. Each of the approximately 200 sutras in the text was his experiential realization, written to effect the same experiential replication in its reader.[3]

—Manoj Kaimal

Why Do We Suffer?

Drastr drsyayoh samyogah heyahetu
Patanjali mentions that the cause of suffering is 'samyoga', the union/ identification between the drastr, *seer and* drasyayoh, *seen (the partner, the job, the image, the house, the cars).*[4]

—Patanjali's *Yoga Sutras*, chapter 2, sutra 17[5]

We seek meaning in relationships, food, frenzied activity, and exercise, besides getting enslaved in other addictive patterns like alcohol, tobacco, drugs—all to fill the void and ease the restlessness in our hearts. So while it is easy to blame other people and situations—'my parents messed up my childhood, my boss is a tyrant, my cholesterol levels are high, my partner stresses me out', ultimately we have to take responsibility for our own lives and the state of our minds.

The onus is on us to do the inner work that is required; through reflection, contemplation and meditation, to make that shift from outer focus to inner focus and connect with ourselves.

So we must earnestly seek that connection with ourselves, and to

3 Manoj Kaimal, *Making Patanjali Palatable* (Manoj Kaimal, 2008).

4 All translations of the verses from the *Yoga Sutras* are the author's own interpretation.

5 'Manasa Yoga' *Teacher Training Notes.*

me there is no greater path to embark on than yoga. Yoga is an inner journey, a process through which our lives evolve and transform. A lot of us also consciously or unconsciously live in the clutches of suffering. As we connect to the essence of the practice, as our awareness deepens, we consciously release patterns that keep us in bondage or do not honour us. So this book rose from my need to share the transformational effect of yoga and the power of the inner connection that I had experienced in my own life with others who are seeking it. It is also about encouraging people to consciously embark on the work necessary to alleviate suffering and find their inner alignment, so that their lives flow like a beautifully choreographed 'vinyasa'—a sequential blending of body, mind, heart and spirit. Therein lies the joy, therein lies the yoga.

The universe communicates with us all the time, but because we are neither tuned into ourselves nor to the world around us, we are not able to decipher its language. But as we do the work, its magic is revealed to us and our paths become guided and illuminated. The word 'educate' etymologically means 'to draw out'. Knowledge and, ultimately, wisdom, have to be drawn out of us so that they can shine forth. It has to be earned from within and be reflected in our actions through our own effort as *shravanam* (hearing), *mananam* (reflection), and *nidhidyasanam* (contemplation). So let us make cultivating our inner connection a priority. When we suffer; when we are upset, anxious, disturbed, agitated or in pain, it is really an invitation for us to look within and explore the cause of our suffering. Inner connection is a conscious seeking, and we cultivate it by deepening our awareness of ourselves—our body, our breath, our thoughts and mental patterns and the world around us. Our asana practice, other sitting meditative practices, journaling, reflecting, contemplating, spending time in nature, all directs us inward. So every day we must put some time aside to strengthen the ultimate relationship of all, the one with ourselves! For when our inner world shifts, like magic, our outer world shifts too.

> *We are what we think.*
> *All that we are arises with our thoughts.*
> *With our thoughts we make the world.*
> *Speak or act with an impure mind*
> *And trouble will follow you*
> *As the wheel follows the ox that draws the cart.*
> *We are what we think.*
> *All that we are arises with our thoughts.*
> *With our thoughts we make the world.*
> *Speak or act with a pure mind*
> *And happiness will follow you*
> *As your shadow, unbreakable.*[6]
>
> —Buddha

Practice

1. Set aside some time for yourself every day. Sit in silence for at least 10 minutes—first thing is the morning is the best. At that time, the mind is relatively clear.
2. Watch your thoughts. View this as a process of getting to know yourself. Who occupies your mind? What occupies your mind? Is there any situation that is troubling you? It will show up.
3. Connect to the tone of your mind. What is the state of your mind? Is it joy? Is it sadness? Is it anguish? Is it inspired? Is it boredom or sleepiness? Is it rage? Whatever it might be,

6 Thomas Byron, *The Dhammapada: The Sayings of the Buddha* (New York: Vintage Books, 2012).

however uncomfortable it might be, witness it, acknowledge it—the anger, the rage, the tears, and the disillusionment. Let it flow, release.

Asanas: Backbends to Open the Heart

When we experience major trauma, the instinctive reaction is to shrink; to want to shut down, to take cover. But on the contrary, the invitation of life and yoga is to keep expanding, to keep evolving. Through back bends, we strive to keep the heart open through the heartbreak and tears, through good times and tough ones.

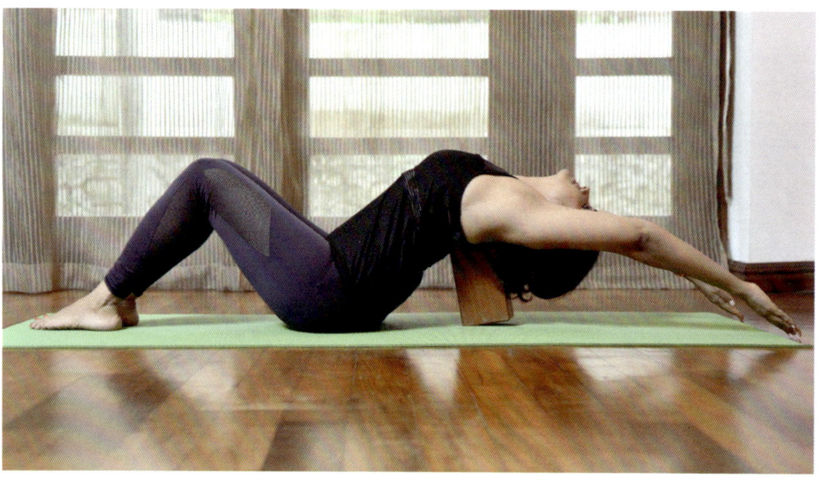

Paryakasana: Couch Pose

1. Sit on the floor, with your legs kept straight in front of you.
2. Place a vertical block behind you. Carefully arch and lower your upper back on the block and hold the position. This gives a nice opening to the upper back.
3. Breathe deeply. Beginners may keep their knees bent feet on the floor (as shown in the picture), as that is easier on the back. They can also place the block horizontally so that the height is lower and the back does not have to arch so deep.

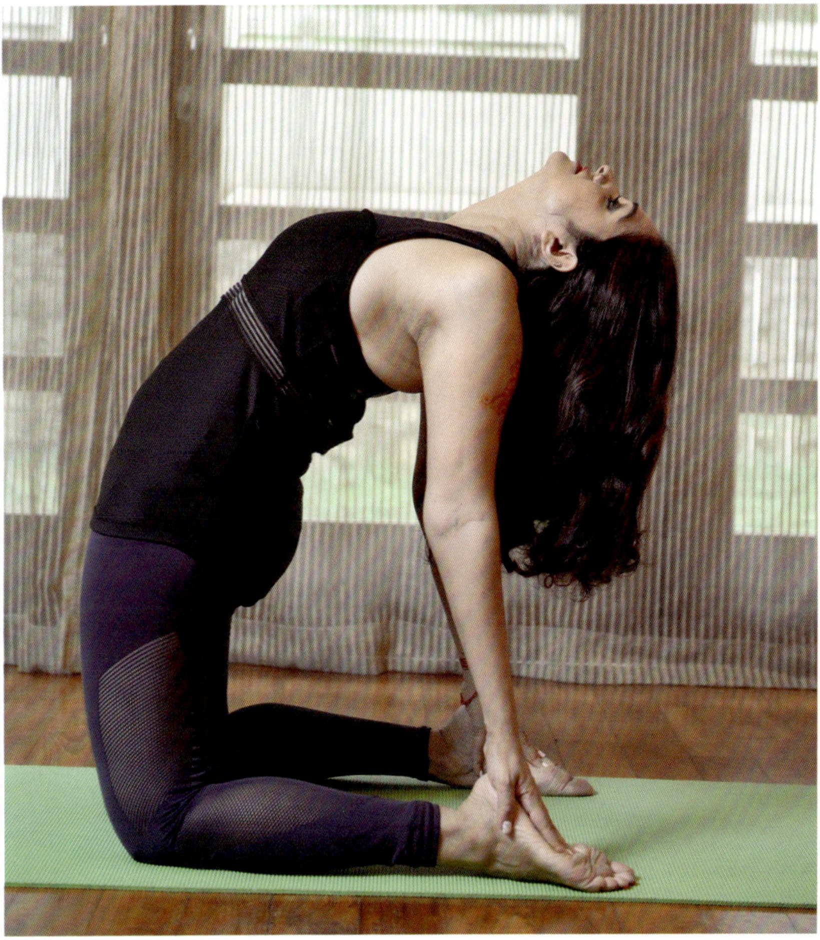

Ustrasana: Camel Pose

1. Stand on your knees and shins. Align your knees and heels to be hip-width apart.

2. Place both hands on your heels and arch back, lifting through the heart, while allowing your pelvis to move forward.

3. Option - Twist a bit to right, and place your right hand on your right heel, lift your left arm up and arch back, allowing your chest to open and pelvis to move forward. This opens the front of your body. Repeat on the other side.

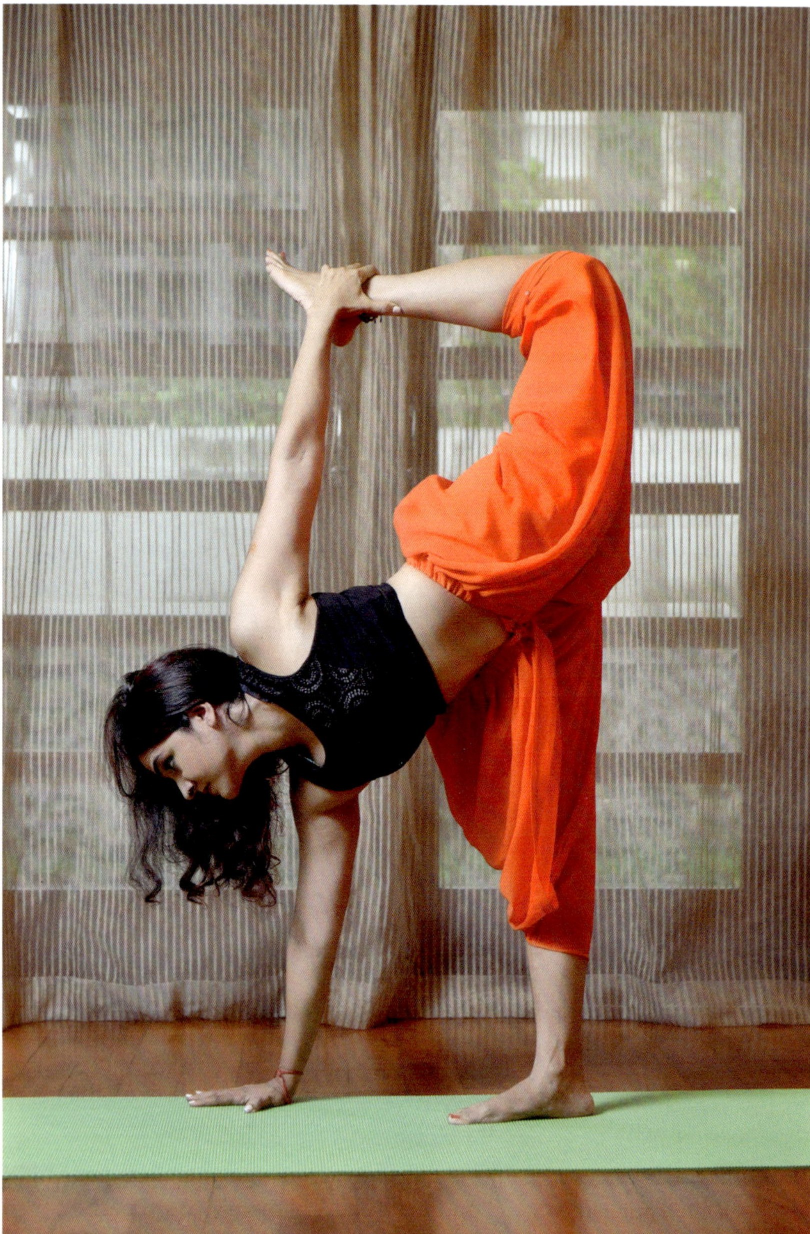

Adhomukha Natarajasana or Downward-Facing Natarajasana (Lord of the Dancers)

Exploring Yoga

As animals, we walk the earth. As bearers of divine essence, we are among the stars. As human beings, we are caught in the middle, seeking to reconcile the paradox of how to make our way upon earth while striving for something more permanent and more profound.[1]

—Guruji B.K.S. Iyengar

Mention the word 'yoga' and it conjures many words and images in our minds. But along with its phenomenal popularity, there are many misconceptions about it. For some of us, yoga is about getting all tied up in knots! For some others it's about getting twisted like a pretzel or contorting their bodies into seemingly impossible positions! In the current age of social media like Facebook and Instagram, yoga has become a path to claim fame; a means to garner attention (read: likes) as they hashtag the spotlight towards their incredibly flexible bodies. Browse #yogasites or follow so-called yogis on Instagram (and there are many, both male and female) and you will be dazzled by

1 B.K.S. Iyengar, *Light on Life: The Yoga Journey to Wholesomeness, Inner Peace, and Ultimate Freedom* (USA: Rodale Inc., 2005).

the incredible number of semi-nude bodies positioned in various poses against breathtakingly beautiful backgrounds. It truly is a feast for the eyes, if you are into appreciating the beauty of nature.

But it doesn't stop there. For some people yoga is a religion, for some others it is a 'cult'. In my experience as a yoga teacher for almost two decades now, I have heard it all: 'I am too young for yoga', 'too old for yoga', 'my body is too stiff'. For some others, yoga is about sitting cross-legged with closed eyes and seeking the elusive 'inner peace'. And then there are so many learned people, spiritual teachers and relatives, who will tell you rather scornfully that Hatha yoga practice is an exercise to keep the body healthy and is therefore somehow inferior, and that learning the scriptures is the true path to evolution. I just see all of this as the play of the ego, which needs to believe that their path is the one true path! However, there is no one true path.

The story of the Blind Men and the Elephant begs to be shared here:

This is a famous Indian tale of six blind men who each came across a different part of the elephant. One of them touched the tusk, another held the trunk and yet another held the ear. The fourth one touched the surface of the body, the fifth held onto the leg and the sixth its tail!

And each of them came away arguing and holding on very strongly to the view that the elephant was limited to the part they had touched. 'The elephant is a pillar, No! It's like a rope, No no! It's like a big hand fan, it's a solid pipe.' Thus each blind man created his own version of reality from his limited experience and perspective, while the truth or reality of the elephant was so much more than each one experienced individually.

In philosophy departments around the world, the story of the Blind Men and the Elephant has become the poster child for moral relativism and religious tolerance.

Similarly, there are the many branches and styles of yoga! A newbie could be forgiven for feeling overwhelmed by the many names and forms of yoga, so here's an attempt to decode it.

The Main Branches of Yoga

Raja Yoga: Raja alludes to the highest state of yoga practice: Samadhi. Subsequently, Swami Vivekananda equated it with the path prescribed in the *Yoga Sutras* of Patanjali. Another ancient text, the *Hatha Yoga Pradipika*, refers to Hatha yoga as the means to achieving Raja yoga.

Karma Yoga: While the traditional translation of 'karma' is action, in the Manasa yoga context, it is also interpreted as movement. And the practice of Karma yoga involves the steady awareness of the different movements of the body, breath and mind. As we keep watching, it begins to dawn on us that the organs of action and perception, including the mind and the intellect, are all functioning independently. The eyes keep seeing, the ears keep hearing, the mind keeps thinking and we realize that this 'I' notion that we have of ourselves has very little to do with any of these body and mind functions. This realization is very humbling as we understand that there is a greater intelligence that flows through us, and this reduces the sense of 'doership' in our actions.

As we continue to observe our movements and actions, we also realize how each action sets forth a sequence of other actions, as we are all interconnected. There cannot be an isolated action. Each action ripples across the fabric of the universe in ways that we cannot fathom. This gives rise to a sense of responsibility in the way we wield our powers of thought, speech and action. And as we recognize our interconnectedness with others, our sense of empathy is enhanced too.

Then we undertake actions which are not only in consideration of our individualistic benefits, but are on a larger universal scale—the benefits of which accrue to more than just 'I, the individual' or 'I, the family'.

The karma yogi consecrates each action to the benefit and in service of the universe at large, at which point karma becomes a yagna, an offering. As the Bhagavad Gita says, everything is an offering to Brahman, by the Brahman—*Brahmaarpanam*.[2]

Jnana Yoga: Jnana stands for wisdom, and therefore, Jnana yoga is the path of studying and contemplating the scriptures and applying it skillfully on a moment-to-moment basis through the choices that we make and the actions that we take.

Bhakti Yoga: Bhakti means devotion. Here we are conscious of a presence larger than ourselves, more complex than we can comprehend, and we practice seeing everyone and the events in our lives in the context of the working of this larger principle.

Hatha Yoga: Hatha yoga is the practice of attaining deep insightful absorption into our energy and consciousness through the use of asana, pranayama, *bandhas*, *mudras* and *kriyas*.

Hatha Yoga is a branch of yoga that emerges from another great philosophical tradition of India called Tantra. Though it is a very loosely used term today, we must know that any practice that involves asana, pranayama, *bandhas*, *mudras*, and *kriyas* falls under the broad umbrella of Hatha Yoga.

Styles of Hatha Yoga

If one goes to a gym or a yoga centre one would be truly amazed at the number of styles of yoga that have emerged over the years. From the traditional classical styles of Sivananda yoga, Iyengar

2 Paramahansa Yoganada, *God Talks With Arjuna: The Bhagavad Gita* (Kolkata: Yagoda Satsanga Society, 2011).

yoga and Ashtanga Vinyasa yoga, we now have Acro yoga, Integral yoga, Hot yoga, Jivamukti yoga, Tantra yoga, Kundalini yoga, Yin yoga, Power yoga, Oscillation yoga etc., to name a few. It doesn't stop there. Then there are the hybrids: yoga and pilates, yoga and martial arts, yoga and flying, yoga and weights, yoga and dance. Now there are even studios offering 'Ganja yoga' and 'Beer yoga!' Need I say more on the myriad styles of yoga?

Is There Any Kind of Right or Wrong Yoga?

First, we must know that yoga is a state of mind, and is not limited to a shape we create with the body. So on the face of it, we could look like we are in *bakasana*, crow pose, but, if in our minds we are lost in comparison and competition with the person next to us, then we are engaged in a purely physical practice of strength.

Hence for the beginner, it is useful to know Patanjali's direction—that yoga is a *shasanam* (discipline). The discipline is to be aware of the mind and its modulations—the need to label, judge, compare, measure, hold on, compete, etc., without getting identified by it, and direct it to be grounded in the 'present'. In yoga class, students are directed to be aware of their bodies, breath and states of mind. With regular practice, the students' consciousness will slowly shift from restlessness and agitation into *ekagra* (the state of one-pointed concentration) and eventually into *niruddha* (dissolution), two states of mind where yoga happens.

Yogacharya Tirumalai Krishnamacharya

Considered the 'Father of Modern Yoga', Yogacharya Tirumalai Krishnamacharya deserves a special mention for keeping the torch of yoga burning bright in recent history. In the beginning of the 20th century, after nearly 400 years of British rule—as there were many regions of India under the rule of the British East India Company from the 1600s—many areas of knowledge systems concerning health and spirituality were destroyed. In these dark times, yoga too faced the ignominy of becoming a forgotten discipline.

Young Krishnamacharya was already an expert in many disciplines including Vedanta, Nyaya, Mimamsa, *Sankhya* and *Vaisesika*. Yet, something deep in him propelled him to study the science of yoga to its greatest depths. He embarked on a long and arduous journey and after two-and-a-half months of walking, he reached the Himalaya Mountains, at the banks of Lake Mansarovar. There he met his guru, Sri Ramamohana Brahmachari, with whom he stayed for seven-and-a-half years and learnt all that was necessary for the chain of learning to continue. His teacher then ordered him to take up the duty of revitalizing yoga. Such was his dedication to his teacher's words that it became his mission in life, and he spent the rest of his life doing just that.

In 1924, Krishnamacharya returned to Mysore, his hometown, to begin the difficult task of restoring yoga to its former glory in the face of fading enthusiasm from the public during the British Raj. Luckily, he found a patron in the King of Mysore, Sri Krishna Rajendra Wadiyar IV. He was a staunch supporter of yoga and its most eminent teacher, Krishnamacharya, and he helped establish the yogasala at his Jaganmohan Palace in Mysore. It was here that Krishnamacharya began his professional yoga career and worked to revive the great tradition of yoga.

He went on to inspire so many modern-day icons of yoga, including Indra Devi, Pattabhi Jois, B.K.S. Iyengar and T.K.V. Desikachar. As *Yoga Journal* succinctly described in an article entitled, 'Krishnamacharya's Legacy':

> *You may never have heard of him, but Tirumalai Krishnamacharya influenced or perhaps even invented your yoga. Whether you*

> *practice the dynamic series of Pattabhi Jois, the refined alignments of B.K.S. Iyengar, the classical postures of Indra Devi, or the customized Vinyasa (of Desikachar), your practice stems from one source: a five-foot, two-inch Brahmin born more than 100 years ago in a small South Indian village.*[3]

Krishnamacharya believed yoga to be 'India's greatest gift to the world'. By developing and refining different approaches, he made it accessible to millions around the world.

Each of Krishnamacharya's students went on to become legends in their own name, and helped make yoga the phenomenally popular practice around the world that it is today. Guruji B.K.S. Iyengar was actually Krishnamacharya's brother-in-law. He was born a very sickly child, and throughout his childhood he was plagued with ill health. But as destiny would have it, when he was around fourteen years of age, he stayed with his sister and became Krishnamacharya's student and the rest, as they say, is history. He went on to become one of the leading lights of yoga in the world and was awarded the Padma Shri in 1991, the Padma Bhushan in 2002 and the Padma Vibhushan in 2014 by the Indian government. In 2004, Iyengar was named one of the 100 most influential people in the world by *Time* magazine. He is credited with introducing the use of straps, wooden blocks, and other objects as aids in achieving the correct postures in yoga.

Guruji Pattabhi Jois popularized the Ashtanga Vinyasa system, where practices like pranayama (breathing practices), *bandhas*, (core muscular and energetic locks) and *dristi* (points where the eyes should focus) along with asanas and vinyasas were used, as taught to him by his guru, Krishnamacharya. Popular yoga styles

---

3 Fernando Pagés Ruiz, 'Krishnamacharya's Legacy', *Yoga Journal*, May/June issue (2011).

such as vinyasa, power, and rocket yoga are all variations derived from the Ashtanga Vinyasa system.

Guruji T.K.V. Desikachar was the son of Krishnamacharya. Desikachar went on to develop a highly personalized approach to yoga that tailors the practice to each student's specific physical condition, emotional state, age, cultural background, and interests. It follows Krishnamacharya's famous maxim: '*Teach what is within you. Not as it applies to you, but as it applies to the one in front of you*'.

Indra Devi, often called 'The First Lady of Yoga', was Russian by birth. Krishnamacharya admitted her into his school only at the behest of the Maharaja of Mysore—making her the first woman *chela* (pupil) and the first Western woman ever at an Indian ashram. She took yoga to Hollywood, counting stars like Gloria Swanson, Greta Garbo, Robert Ryan, violinist Yehudi Menuhin etc., as her students. In Shanghai, she taught what was believed to be the first yoga class in modern China. She was also credited with lifting the ban on yoga in Russia after the communist revolution, and publishing the country's first book on yoga.

Of course this list is incomplete, and there are many other famous yoga gurus known and unknown who, over the years, have kept the flame of yoga burning bright with their own unique understanding and offering to the fires of yoga. Swami Sivananda Saraswati (Sivananda Yoga Vedanta Centers), Maharishi Mahesh Yogi (Transcendental Meditation Movement), Swami Satyananda Saraswati (Bihar School of Yoga), Swami Satchidananda (Integral Yoga) and Paramahansa Yogananda (Self-Realization Fellowship, Kriya Yoga) are a few of the giants of the past. Today, Sri Sri Ravi Shankar (Art of Living Foundation), Baba Ramdev (Patanjali Yogpeeth), H.H. Pujya Swami Chidanand Saraswatiji (Parmarth Niketan), and Sadhguru (Isha Foundation) are some names that continue to make yoga waves the world over.

Is Yoga a Class?

It is very common to hear people talk about attending a yoga class once or twice a week. So the question arises, 'Is the practice of yoga limited to a class?' While 'yoga class' is just a general term commonly used for convenience, it is important to know that yoga is not limited to a class. Different scriptures have different definitions of yoga. In the *Yoga Sutras*, Patanjali prescribes 'Ashtanga yoga', the eight-step path with the culmination being the state of samadhi or absorption. Another famous commentator of the sutras, Sage Vyasa, too says yoga is 'samadhi'. In the Bhagavad Gita, one very popular definition is '*Yoga karmasu kaushalam*', i.e., yoga is skillful action. Another popular line from a verse in the Gita is, '*Samatvam yoga uchyate*', the evenness of the mind is yoga.[4]

According to Manoj Kaimal, yoga is for 'darshanam'—clear, insightful seeing. Initially, as we begin the practice with our limited vision, we connect to the body at a superficial level—as muscle, tissues and bone. But as our vision improves, we begin to connect to the more subtle layers of the body—as energy, lightness, spaciousness and vibration. Similarly, as beginners we get caught up in the grossness of the movement of the body, as shapes etc.

But again, as our vision improves, as our ability to see becomes clearer, we begin to explore the questions, 'Who is orchestrating the movement of our arms?', 'Who is moving our leg back into lunge position?', or 'Who is doing the down dog position?' And we begin to connect not just to the seen—the shapes, the words, the form etc., but also to the intangible intelligent presence that enlivens the body. Thus the practice of asana becomes an experiential 'darshanam', of not just seeing the body, but of experiencing our greater self.

---

4 Paramahansa Yogananda, *God Talks With Arjuna: The Bhagavad Gita* (Kolkata: Yagoda Satsanga Society of India, 2011).

Guruji B.K.S. Iyengar, in his book *Light on the Yoga Sutras of Patanjali*, says:

> *Darsana means 'vision of the soul' and also 'mirror'. The practice of yoga is to reflect the thoughts and actions of the aspirant as in a mirror. The practitioner observes the reflections of his thoughts, mind, consciousness and actions, and corrects himself. The process guides him towards observation of his inner self.* [5]

Thus while our mat practice may end with class, our yoga practice, as awareness practice, continues throughout the day.

Practice

1. Be aware of your body, your feet and other sensations for the first few minutes after waking up. Be aware of the sensation of solidity when your feet touch the floor as you get out of bed and take a few steps.
2. Try and sense energy as you walk, do your asana practice or engage in any other form of movement.
3. Like the way you watch a movie on a screen, practice witnessing your mind, seeing your thoughts, as well as the different characters and drama that accompany it. This helps you connect to your witnessing capacity—the seer, and, with time, become less identified and enmeshed with the seen.

Asana: *Surya Namaskar*, or Sun Salutations

The sun salutation practice directs us to connect to the light and energy within us, the embodiment of light and energy that we are. Each movement is made with an awareness of the energy behind the movement of the arms and legs.

5 B.K.S. Iyengar, *Light on the Yoga Sutras of Patanjali* (London: Thorsons, 1993).

1. Place your palms in Namaste.

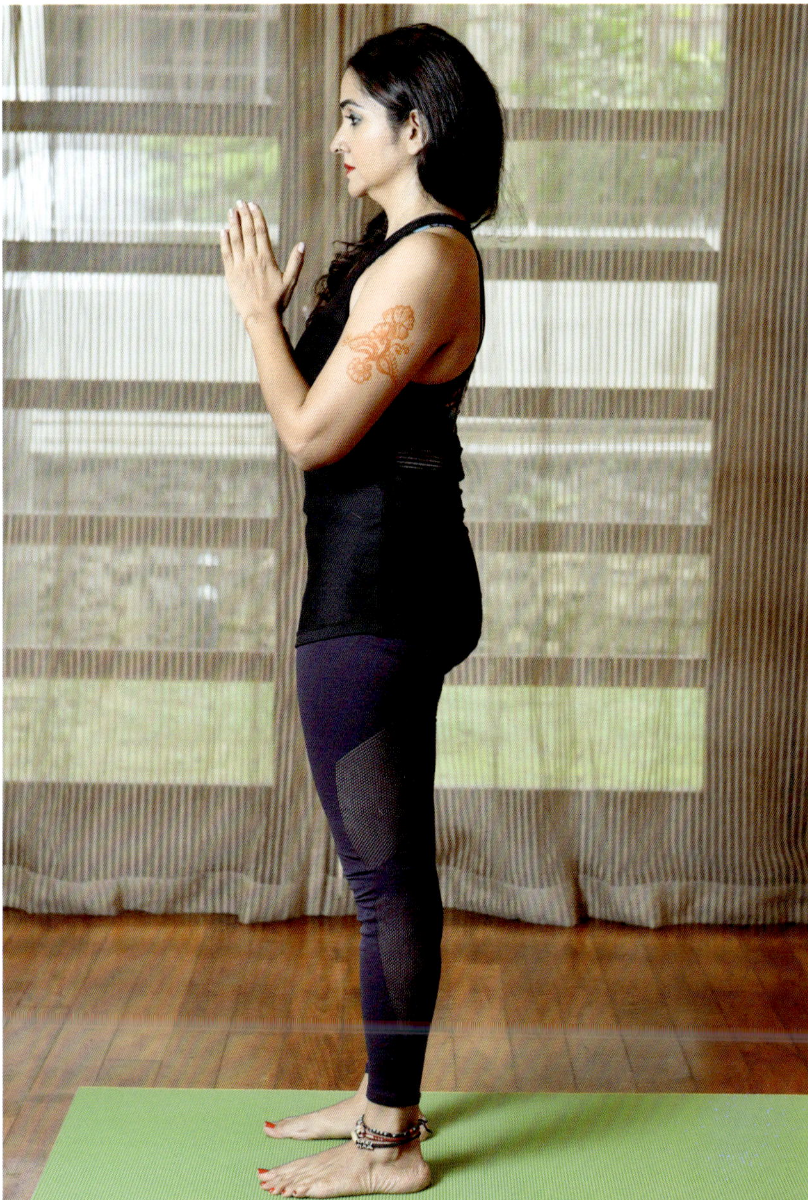

2. Inhale, open your chest, draw the front of your pelvis upward towards your chest and arch back, raising your arms upward and backward.

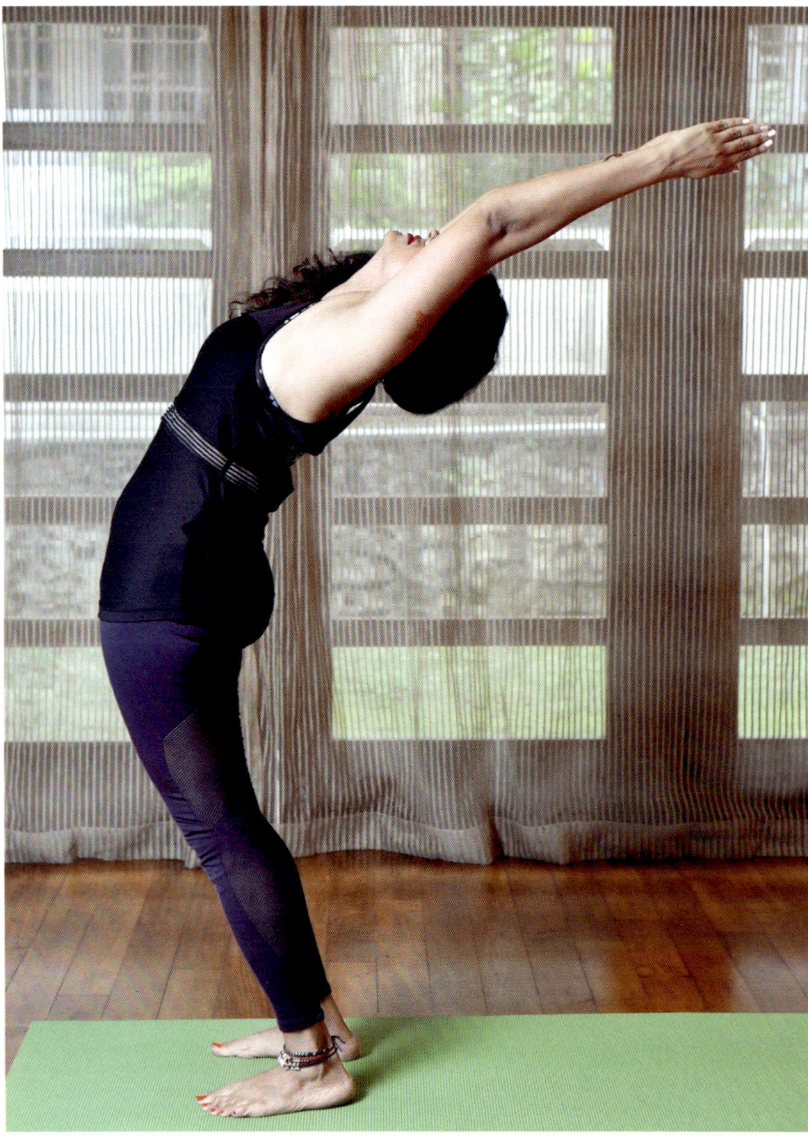

3. Exhale, tip your pelvis forward, and lower your hands towards the floor. You can bend your knees if necessary.

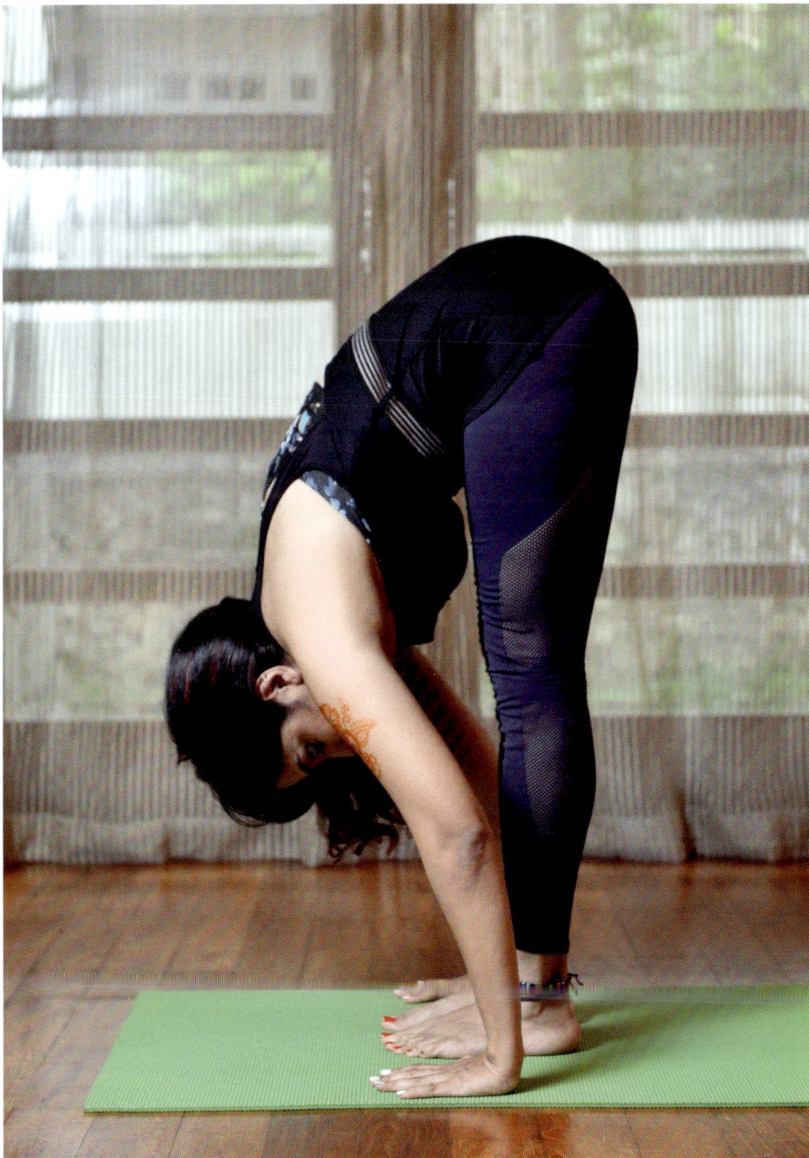

4. Inhale, take a step back with your right leg, and lower your knee onto the floor with your foot pointed backward. Keep your chest open and lift the heart as you look forward.

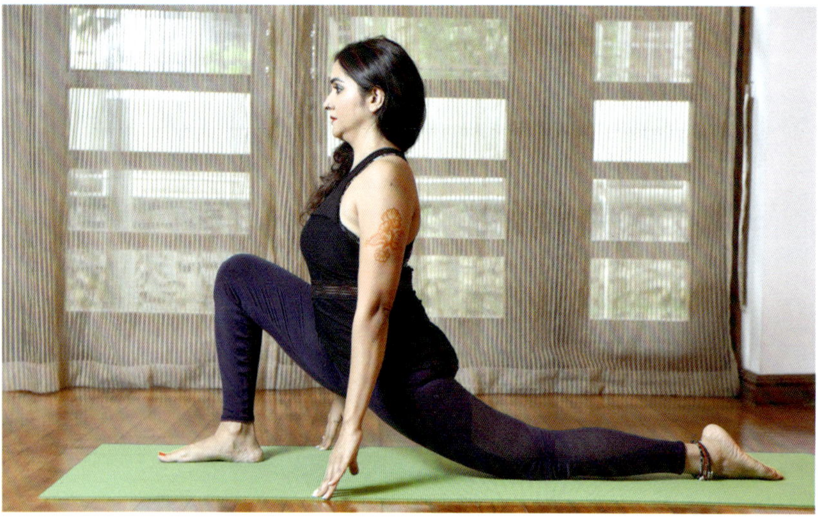

5. Retain your breath, and take a step back with your left leg into plank position.

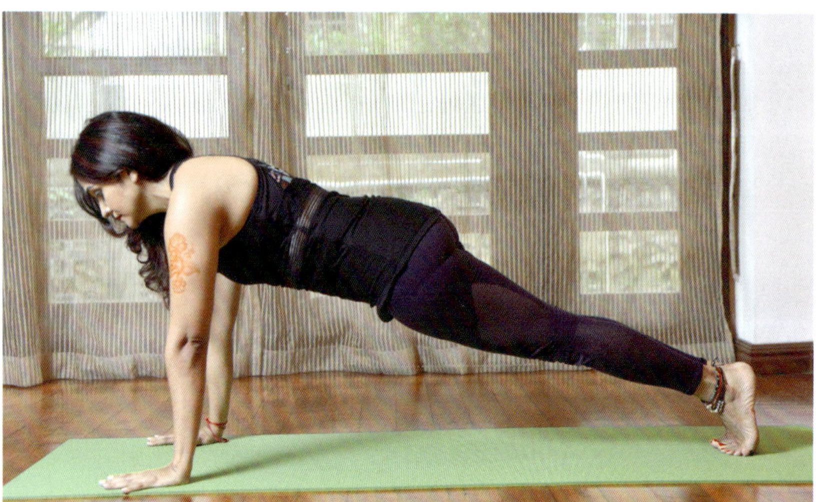

6. Exhale, and lower your knees, chest and chin onto the floor.

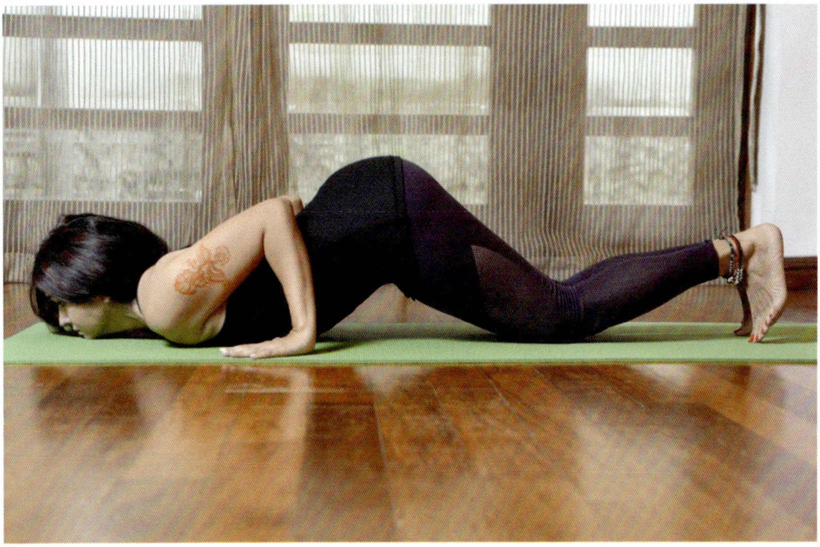

7. Inhale, lower your hips, straighten your arms and arch back into cobra position.

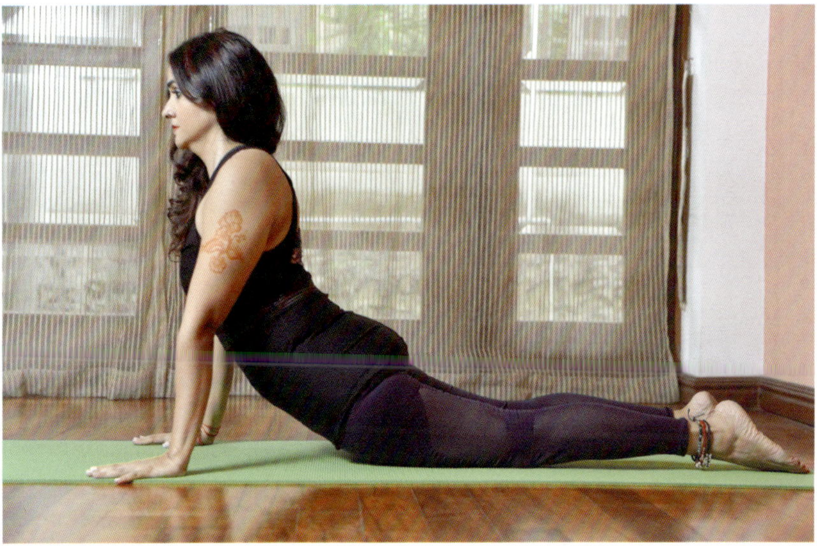

8. Exhale, press down through your palms and lift your hips up and back into downward-facing dog position.

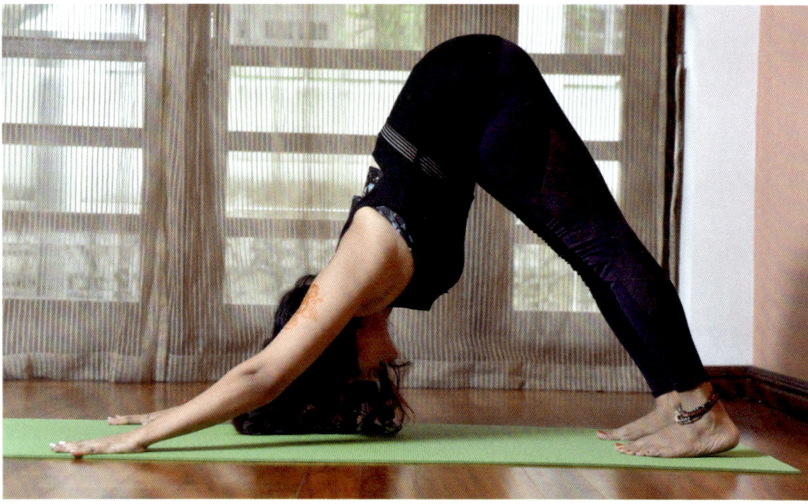

9. Inhale, take a step forward with your right foot, between your hands if possible.

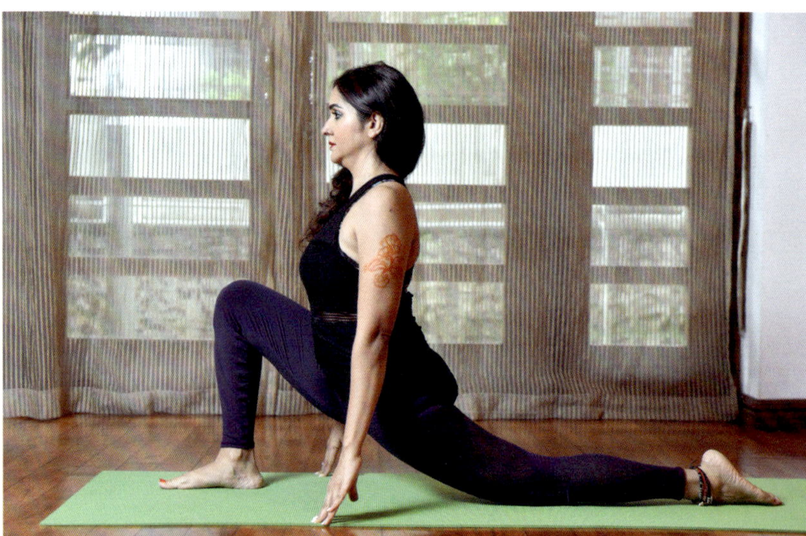

10. Exhale, take a step forward with your left leg into the standing forward fold.

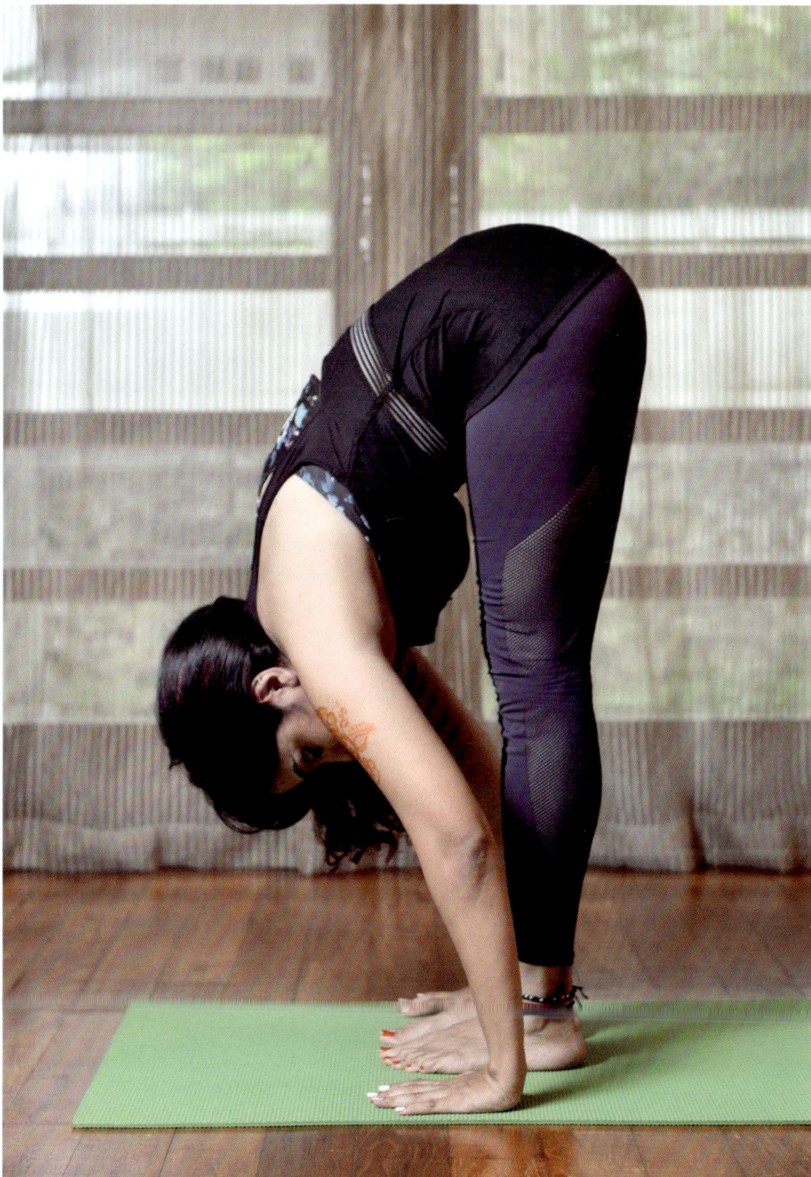

11. Inhale, lift your arms up and arch back.

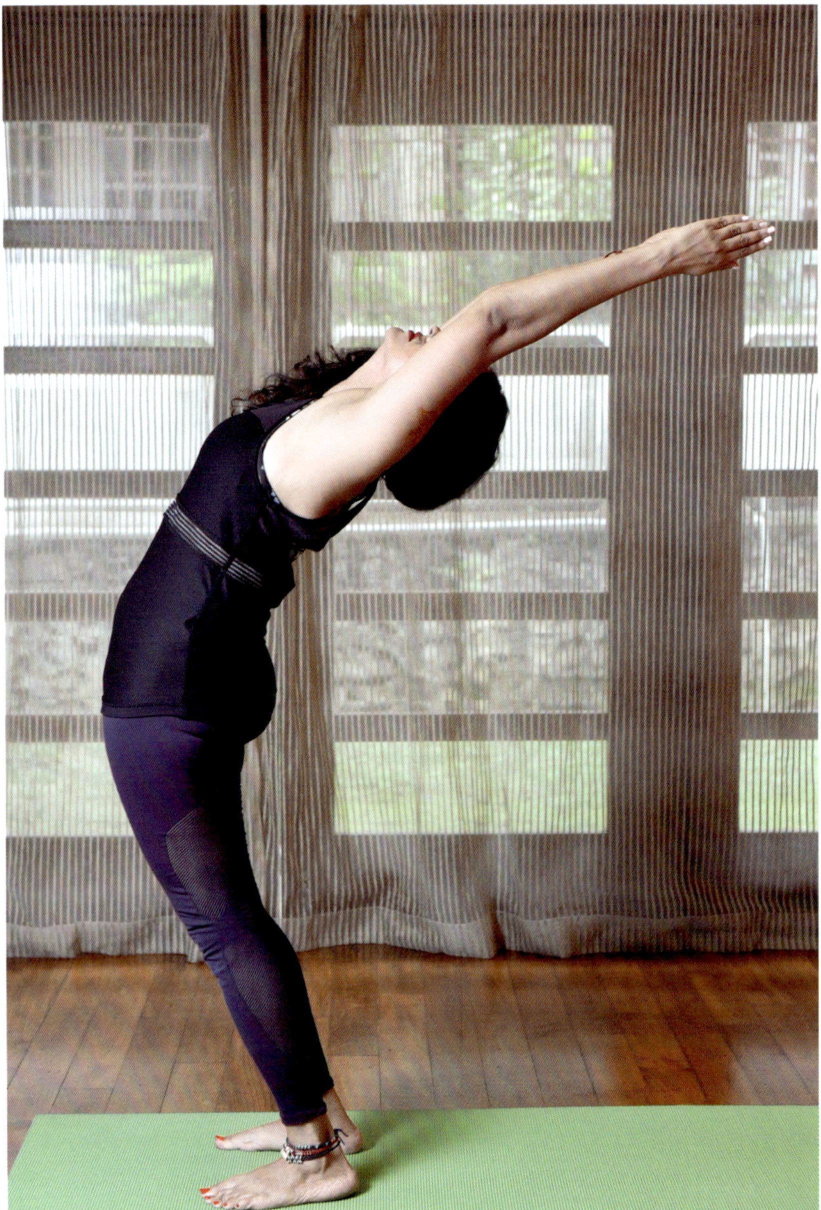

12. Exhale, lower your arms down by your side.

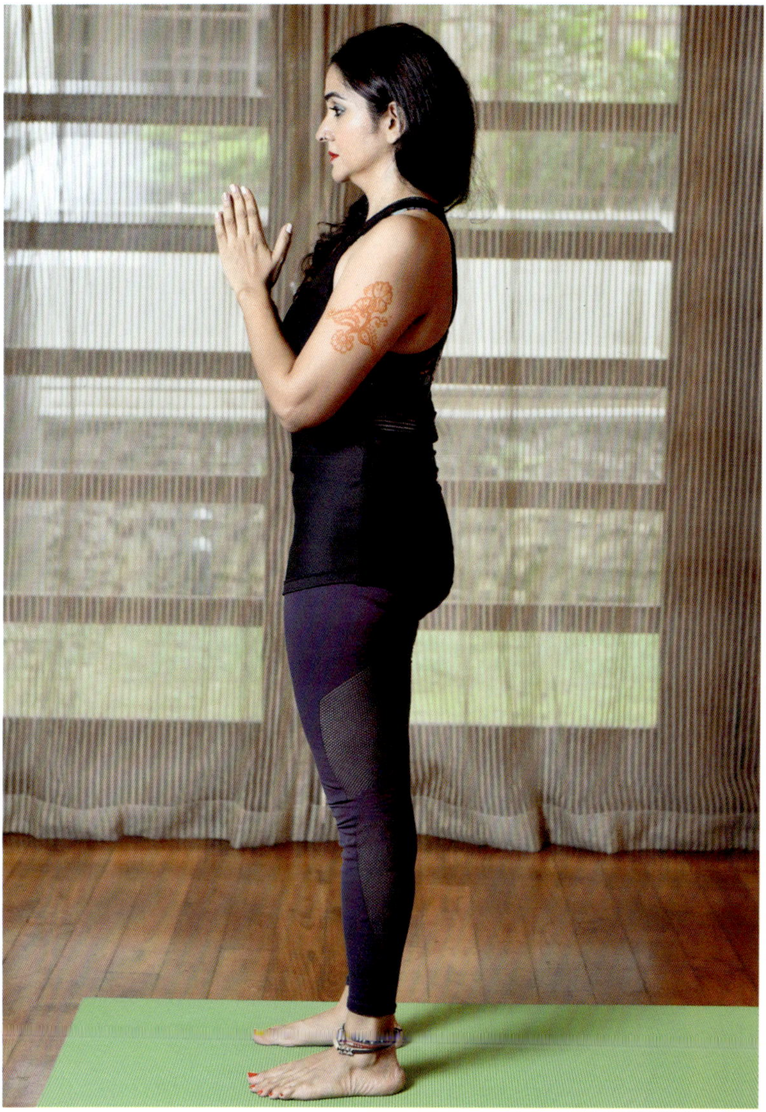

Repeat with your left leg going back in the third position, and your left leg going forward in the ninth position.

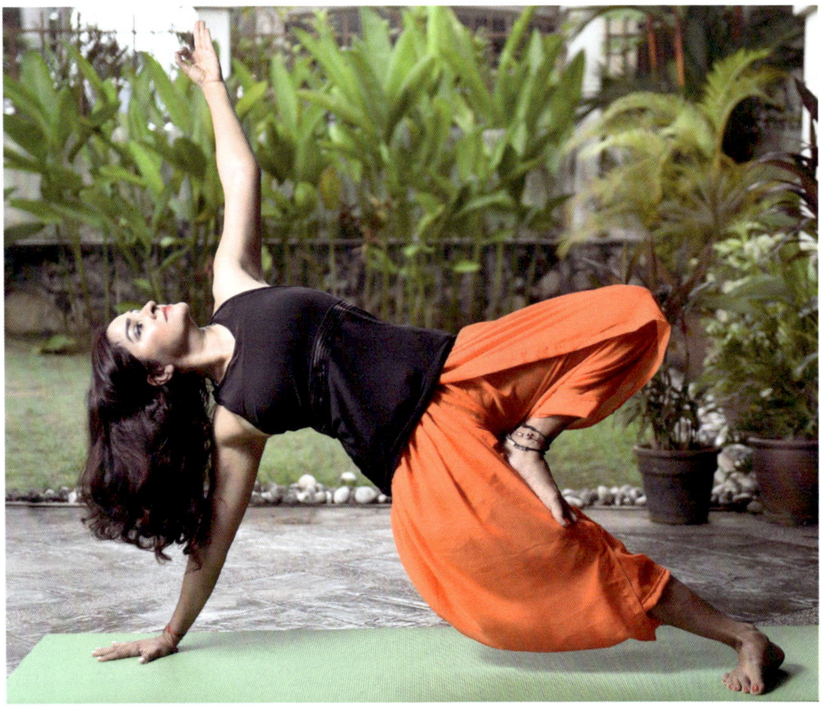

Artistic Pose: *Vasistavrksasana*

Awareness

'Gnothi Seauton: Know Thyself'
This ancient Greek aphorism is one of the Delphic Maxims inscribed in the pronaos (forecourt) of the temple of Apollo at Delphi, the site of the sacred Oracle.

The path of yoga is transformative, and transformation begins with awareness. We have to know ourselves: what are our thoughts? What are our patterns? What are our intentions and motivations? What causes us to act? What causes us to react? What are our triggers and irritants? If we are not aware of what we are thinking or how we are acting, then there is little chance for us to break the pattern of our thoughts and actions and do things differently.

'Awareness precedes change. You will never be able to eliminate a weakness you don't even know about!'[1]

—Robin Sharma

1 Robin Sharma, *Who Will Cry When You Die?* (Mumbai: Jaico Publishing House, 2009).

The Tyranny of Patterns

Human beings generally operate on patterns. If we take a step back and observe our lives, it will become clear that a lot of our patterns, including eating, exercising, communicating and even thinking, arise not from any great wisdom but from the tight grip of almost-compulsive patterns. The treachery of patterns is that it holds us mindless in our comfort zones, even as it takes us steadily downhill. Despite suffering deeply, we hold on for dear life as we do not want to, or sometimes are simply unable to summon the strength required to make hard but necessary shifts in our lives.

Take the example of a diabetic with a craving for sweets, who will still eat sweets after every meal despite the consequences! Or a woman who is treated without respect in a relationship, but still clings to it because of the established pattern of the relationship. Or an obese person who, despite being advised to lose weight, is still not motivated to make an effort to exercise or change his lifestyle. Or a person who has fits of uncontrolled rage but will not assume responsibility for the physical or verbal abuse, nor take steps to control it. There are numerous instances around us but we need to be able to 'see' it first before we can make any attempt to transform it. Thus, awareness is the first step to transformation.

It does not mean that all patterns are negative or that we need to live without patterns. There is a comfort and a stability to patterns that lends a sense of security to our lives. The focus here is on awareness. We must be aware of what they are. One of the greatest aspects of the practice of yoga is that our level of awareness and sensitivity to ourselves and everything around us deepens and we become more conscious. This begins with the body.

Asana is Life

When my students first come to my class, it is very interesting to note that left hand, right hand, left leg, right leg are all a jumble. They are almost like children trying to figure out left from right! And as I call out to them, asking them to be aware of the direction of their toes and their knees, I can almost see their minds busy scrambling, trying to make sense of my words and connect with them! This is because our bodies and minds are so disconnected.

Through the regular practice of asana, we become more aware of our bodies, breaths and minds. The neural networks get established, leading to greater mind-body coordination and flow. As we talk about awareness in an asana, it means we should be able to direct and hold attention on the body. Then the whole practice of asana becomes a dynamic and creative expression of the flow of energy. Without the element of attention, it remains a repetitive, mechanical, ego-centered practice—about who can find balance in *shirsasana* (head stand) first in class or who can plank longer. Or who can bind in *parsvakonasana* (lateral angle pose) or who can do the perfect spilt in *hanumanasana* (front split).

Awareness of Mind

In class, students are encouraged to cultivate awareness of not just their bodies, but also of the taste of their minds and their emotions, whether it is the feeling of satisfaction at rising into *urdhvadhanurasana* (upward bow pose) or the feeling of dissatisfaction at being unable to touch their toes in *uttanasna* (standing forward fold)! They are directed to be objectively conscious and non-judgmental at the rising of joy and the lightness in their bodies at the end of class, as well as the critical denouncement of the mind on coming face-to-face with stiffness and resistance in a back bend. To sense the expansiveness in the mind as we draw back through the arm bones and keep the heart and chest open, and to taste the disappointment and sadness as our chest closes and shoulders round.

It is important that we see it all—the darkness and the light, the disappointment and the elation, the reactivity of the mind as well as its equanimity, as body and breath flow together in harmony. We need to be aware of how we tend to look around the class and compare ourselves with others, whether we give up easily or we try relentlessly; whether we are critical in the conversations in our head if we don't 'get' an asana, or we are supportive and encouraging of ourselves! We can be our own harshest critics: 'I've been doing this for so long but I still can't get it! My body is stiff as a board, there's no point to this! Everybody can get it except me!', and it's important that we see it all.

It is the same attitudes that we express in yoga class that we hold in life too. I always tell my students that, 'the most important conversation that we have in our lives is the one inside our heads!' With time, this deepening awareness permeates beyond the mat and into our everyday lives, lending us deeper insights into our motivations and actions. We can be sure that if we are comparing and competing with the person next to us in class, we will have the same mindset towards a colleague or a neighbor. If we are harsh and critical towards ourselves when we face resistance in a pose, say, we cannot touch our toes in *paschimotanasana* (seated forward bend) or we fail to lift into *sarvangasana* (shoulder stand), we will have the same attitude when we face resistance in life as well, when things do not go according to our plans, when someone says 'No!' to us. So, through deepening awareness, class becomes a learning ground, and asana practice, a tool of *swadhyaya* or self-study, leading to a deeper understanding of the way our minds operate.

Awareness Precedes Transformation

Only when we know where we stand in terms of any aspect of our lives—be it our diet, exercise patterns, sleep patterns, work patterns, patience levels, or relationship comfort, can we take steps to evolve and transform, if that is what is called for. We tend to 'carry on' or 'settle' because we do not want to upset the apple cart. We would rather not face our greatest fears, lose our job, move across the country, be alone, or accept that we have made some bad choices with regard to health and lifestyle, as we are hesitant to step into the great unknown.

But, in order to take decisive action to release ourselves from the situation and create the life we seek, we must first be conscious and acknowledge our current unhappiness and frustration—the inability of the job or the relationship to provide the satisfaction that we seek, that we are grossly overweight and it seriously affects our health and quality of life, that we are in the grip of alcoholic patterns that are taking us downhill. Only once that is seen, can the rest follow.

The Practice

Thus the practice is to be able to observe/witness without judgment, without labeling and categorizing based on the conditioning and preconceived notions of the mind. As we observe the gyrations of the mind, we become aware of the continuous labeling process of 'good', 'bad', 'like', 'dislike', 'moral', and 'immoral'—a continuous process of judgment that creates only unhappiness and agitation.

By releasing the judgment and labeling, we step out of its resistance patterns and get a taste of the present moment, which is full of possibilities. With it comes the all-important ability to shape the moment in the manner we desire. Thus, by sifting through our thoughts, we develop the power to create the lives we seek. Slowly, this awareness transforms into insight, ideas, clarity, opportunities and inspired action.

Synchronicity

As our awareness deepens, our intuitive capacities begin to deepen as well. We are able to decipher the subtle messages and directions of the universe. The more in-tune we are with the working of the universe, the more synchronicity shows up in our lives and there is an ease and flow to it.

About a year ago, my yoga studio was in the process of shifting to a new home. I was very hesitant about the whole move initially because my husband now lives and works in China and I am still not very fluent in Bahasa Malaysia. But the more I stand back and observe, I am simply amazed at the ease with which the whole process unfolded. From finding a space almost next door, to finding a reliable contractor and getting the whole process of renovation and shifting underway, to having a graffiti artist sent to me and other people show up to help me shape the studio of my dreams; there is an underlying sense of ease, a sense of flow, like it was all meant to be, a part of a greater plan.

> *Around us, life bursts with miracles–a glass of water, a ray of sunshine, a leaf, a caterpillar, a flower, laughter, raindrops. If you live in awareness, it is easy to see miracles everywhere. Each human being is a multiplicity of miracles. Eyes that see thousands of colors, shapes, and forms; ears that hear a bee flying or a thunderclap; a brain that ponders a speck of dust as easily as the entire cosmos; a heart that beats in rhythm with the heartbeat of all beings. When we are tired and feel discouraged by life's*

daily struggles, we may not notice these miracles, but they are always there.[2]

—Thich Nhat Hanh

Practice

1. Bring consciousness into everyday acts—while chewing your food, while lazing in front of the TV, when opening the fridge and reaching for a piece of chocolate!
2. Be in touch with your feelings and emotions. Acknowledge them, however painful or 'that's not me' it may be—humiliation, jealously, envy, hatred, greed. See it all. The ability to simply witness is the saving grace that puts some space and loosens the grip of the emotion.
3. Connect to nature. Be aware of the solidity of earth, the vastness of the sky, the aliveness of the trees, the energy of the waves, the stillness of the mountains.

Asanas: Balance

From a yogic perspective, the state of our bodies and the state of our lives are interconnected. Thus, balance in the body is the foundation for balance in life. Balancing poses are especially challenging as they demand deep attention and also strengthen the foundation we stand on.

2 Thich Nhat Hanh, *Essential Writings* (New York: Orbis Books, 2001).

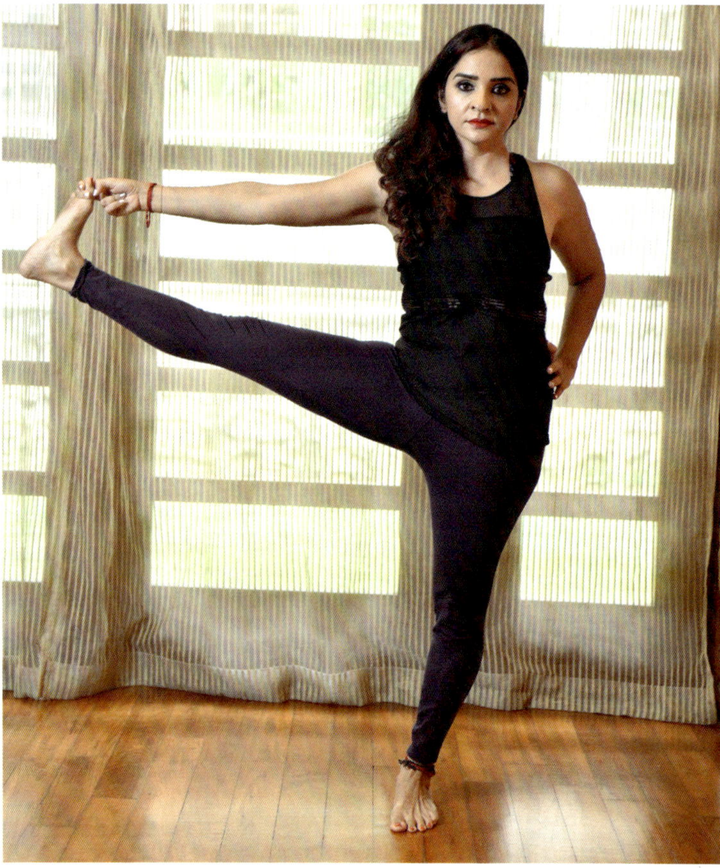

Parsva Utthita Hasta Padangustasana:
Sideways Extended Hand-to-Toe Pose

1. Stand with your feet hip-width apart. Inhale, take your right knee towards your chest and catch hold of the big toe on your right foot, or a strap looped around your foot. Open your knee to the right side.
2. Exhale as you extend your leg out gently to the side as much as possible.
3. Lift through the heart, ground through your left foot, and extend through your right foot, standing tall and broad. Ensure that your navel faces forward.

Repeat on the other side.

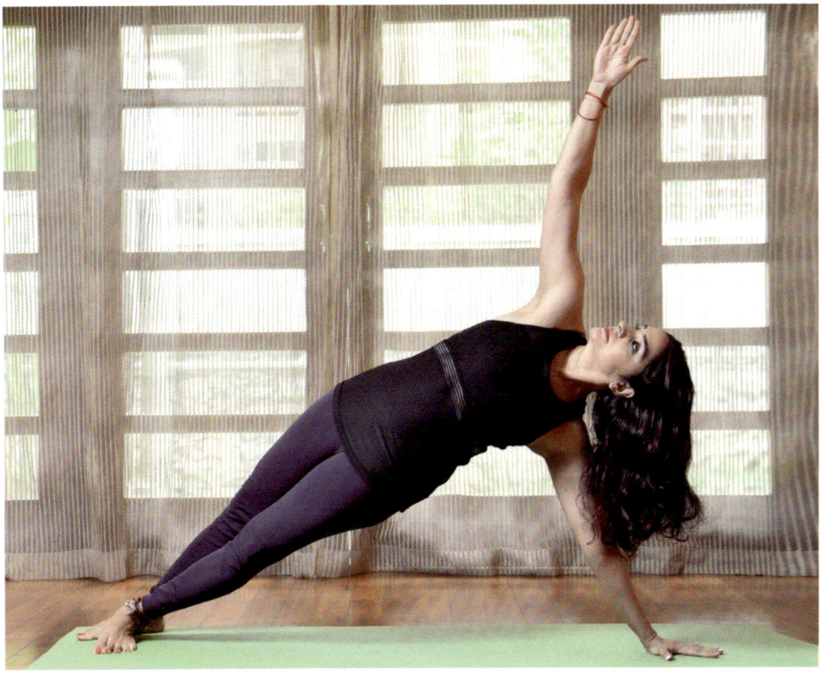

Vasistasana: Side Plank

1. Come in to a plank position. Keep your upper back lifted and tailbone down.
2. Shift your weight to your right hand, take your left arm upward and look up. Keep the front of the torso spinning upward and away from your right arm.
3. Keep your right hip lifted all the time.

Repeat on the other side.

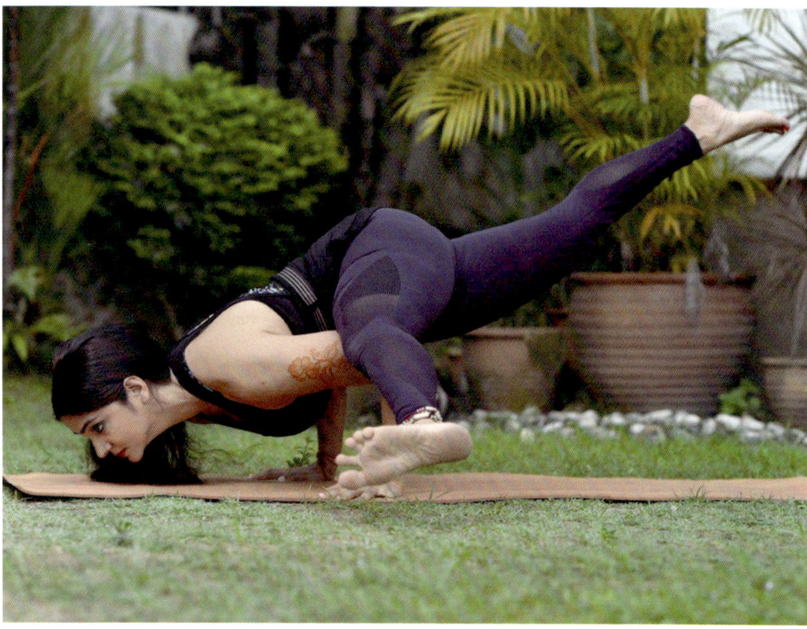

Artistic Pose: *Eka Pada Koundinyasana 2*

Atha: Being in the Now

When you are washing the dishes, washing the dishes must be the most important thing in your life. Just as when you are drinking tea, drinking tea must be the most important thing in your life. Drink your tea slowly and reverently, as if it is the axis on which the whole world revolves — slowly, evenly, without rushing toward the future. Live the actual moment. Only this actual moment is life.

—Thich Nhat Hanh[1]

1 Thich Nhat Hanh, *The Miracle of Mindfulness: The Classic Guide to Meditation by the World's Most Revered Master* (London: Rider Books, 2009).

Yoga is both an ancient, as well as an ever-evolving practice in the 'Now'. The concept of the 'Now' is the key to transformation. Eckhart Tolle wrote a New York Times bestseller with his book *The Power of Now* and made the 'Now' a watchword for a whole generation of people. But long before that, Patanjali wrote about it in his *Yoga Sutras*. In fact, the first word of the first sutra begins with the word *atha—'atha yoga anushasanam'*

So, the practice of yoga is the practice of being in the 'now', in the experience of the currently-unfolding moment.

An untrained mind is always lost in memories, anxieties or in future-based imaginations. In yoga practice, we use the body to anchor the mind to the present. Why the body you may ask? Because the body always operates in the present, it is tangible; you can touch it, feel its solidity, its earthiness, and thus, it is easier to connect with. In the style that I teach, Manasa yoga, each class begins with an *atha* practice. When we come into class, our mind is caught up in different experiences—a traffic jam, a fight with the boss, an altercation with a colleague, an argument with a child etc. The thrust of the practice is, therefore, to shift our awareness from these patterns of thought that consume our mind, and ground it into the body. This grounding or centering happens through directing the student's mind over 16 specific points in the body. By the end of this practice, there is a shift in the mind from the usual ground of story consciousness to the ground of present-moment consciousness.

Our minds are the experiencing capacity of consciousness. Usually our minds are so caught up in the likes and dislikes of an experience that the shifting of the consciousness to the body elicits a deep release from the vice-like grip of the patterns of thought.

As awareness sits on buddhi, intellect, it now guides the mind to take a seat on the experience of the body. And when that happens, our consciousness too shifts from restlessness, agitation and reactivity to a more even, grounded state. The practice of connecting to different points in the body, body sensations, also allows for the activation of insula, the part of the brain that is responsible for feelings of empathy.[1]

—Manoj Kaimal

Atha and Asana

Through asana practice, we abide in not just the physicality of our bodies, but in the presence that we are, as awareness. In asana, the intellect guides the mind to flow through specific anatomical points and lines in the body, to focus on the breath, to be aware of our thoughts. Asana then becomes a beautiful tool to receive the taste of consciousness, to experience the formless. Thus, asana in its fullest, highest sense (not the stretching and gyrations of the body that we have reduced it to), is a portal through which we connect to the body as an experiential throb of energy (*spanda*) of the universe.

In chapter 2, sutra 47 of the *Yoga Sutras,* Patanjali says:

Prayatna shaitilyam ananta samapathibhyam
As we enter the form of the asana, the effort relaxes and in that state of effortless effort, the mind gets absorbed in the Infinite.[2]

---

1 Quotes by Manoj Kaimal, unless specifically cited otherwise, are taken from the Manasa Yoga Teacher Training Notes.

2 'Manasa Yoga' *Teacher Training Notes.*

> *Prayatna (specific efforts) are initially put in with regards to the form of the asana, which steadies the usually unsteady rajas (the guna which stands for movement); and once the energy of rajas is steady, then sattva (the guna that stands for awareness) shaitilyam (releases) its focus on the form, and senses the ananta (limitless) source of its own light, and a samapatti (coalescence) of the form and the formless occurs.*
>
> —Manoj Kaimal

Atha and Life

Like in asana, in the rest of life too, the practice of being present is vital to enhance the quality of our life. Why? Because life is lived and experienced in the present moment. What is life? Life is what is termed, *anubhava dhara*, a flow of experiences. Through the entirety of our lives, we flow seamlessly from one experience to another. As I type, I am having a writing experience, and, as you try to make sense of my words, you are having a reading experience! In fact, the quality of our lives is directly related to the proportion in which our minds are present in our currently unfolding experience. Like beads strung together to create a beautiful necklace, our every experience is strung together to create a memorable lifetime. But the beauty, the depth, the subtleties and intricacies of life can only be experienced if our minds are present in the moment. If our minds are always lost in memories of the past or anxieties of the future, then the present moment, which offers us the only opportunity to drink deeply into the experience of life, is completely lost to us.

The example I always use in class is the morning drive I make with my older son, Vyshnav, every day. If my mind is lost in 'I hate waking up early every morning', or 'I so completely dread this chore, when will I be able to stop doing this?', then I am not being present to the opportunity to share some time with my son. In the process, I too lose out on the wonderful opportunity to engage in a meaningful conversation, share some laughter and create a beautiful lasting memory. Technology does not help, as our unconscious minds have become slaves to it. These days, at least here in Malaysia, it is very common to see four members in a family—parents and two children—out to dinner, ostensibly together, but each lost in their own gadgets. They may be physically in the same place but mentally miles apart, and with different people too! So to put it succinctly, like I teach my kids in their class: 'Wherever your body is, take your mind there too'. It just comes down to that.

So wherever you may be—be it watching a beautiful sunset, driving your child to school, writing, sharing dinner with your family or having chai with a friend, be present to the experience, drink deeply from its depths, taste the joy that each experience offers. Thus we transcend the mundane 'is and was-ness' of everyday life and experience the transcendental 'is' here and now.

We have to realize deeply that the 'Present Moment' is all we ever have. We have to make the 'Now' the primary focus of our lives. The richness and depth of life is in the 'Now'. The sacredness and the mystery, the teaching and the learning, all lie in the 'Now'.

It is vital to be aware of the nature of our minds and its dysfunctions—through its compulsive thought patterns and behavioural manifestations—in order for transformation to happen.

So while walking or climbing, focus on the sensation of touch as your feet hit the ground. You can also use a counting aid to help you remain rooted in the process of walking. Or you can observe your breath with the aid of labels—inhale, exhale etc., to keep your mind stable on your breath. During asana practice, use the tools of your body and your breath to remain grounded in the present.

When you are able to observe your mind, you are no longer trapped in it. You will then begin to connect with something far more powerful: the still, observing 'presence' behind the content of your mind, the grahitir *or observer.*

What is the Ground of Your Consciousness?

So from time to time during the day it is important that we ask ourselves, what are the grounds of our consciousness right now? Acknowledge it even if the grounds are anxiety, fear, hatred, sadness, jealousy or envy. Whatever we may like to think of ourselves, Patanjali explains in the *Yoga Sutras* that we all have the seeds of these emotions in us. They may just be *udharanam* (expressed) or *prasuppta* (dormant). Through my own life experiences I have come to realize that it is in different times of our lives, under different circumstances and on meeting different people, that these different emotions are evoked in us. So it is important to be aware, to not be lulled into some false sense of superiority or become judgmental when we see other people struggling with these emotions. Our minds like to be one-up on people and think 'I would never act like that, or I would never say such things'. But if we had walked in the shoes of that person, if we were in that same desperate situation, in those most compelling circumstances, we never know how we would respond.

In chapter 2, verse 50 of the Bhagavad Gita, yoga is defined as *yoga karmasu kaushalam* or 'skillfulness in action'.[3] Being present to

3 Paramhansa Yogananda, *God Talks With Arjuna: The Bhagavad Gita* (Kolkata: Yagoda Satsanga Society of India, 2011).

life also gives us the opportunity to make each moment skilful, to make conscious choices and thus steer our lives in the direction we choose.

Thus, the ultimate yoga is not just about the alignment of our body but the alignment of our minds to the universal intelligence, so that our lives flow out as a perfectly synchronized symphony.

Practice

1. As you climb the staircase in your house, be present to every step you take. Really connect to the sensation of your feet against the floor.
2. As you exercise on the treadmill or stepper, be present to the sensation of the soles of your feet on the machine, to the movement of your legs and arms. Try and coordinate it with your breath so that body and breath flow in harmony.
3. As you type on the computer, be present to the sensation of your fingers flowing across the keyboard, and the touch of your fingers on the mouse.

Asana: Strength

Strength is a core aspect of asana practice as it is in life. As our minds and bodies are seamless, connecting to our capacity for strength in asana connects us to our inner strength and draws it out.

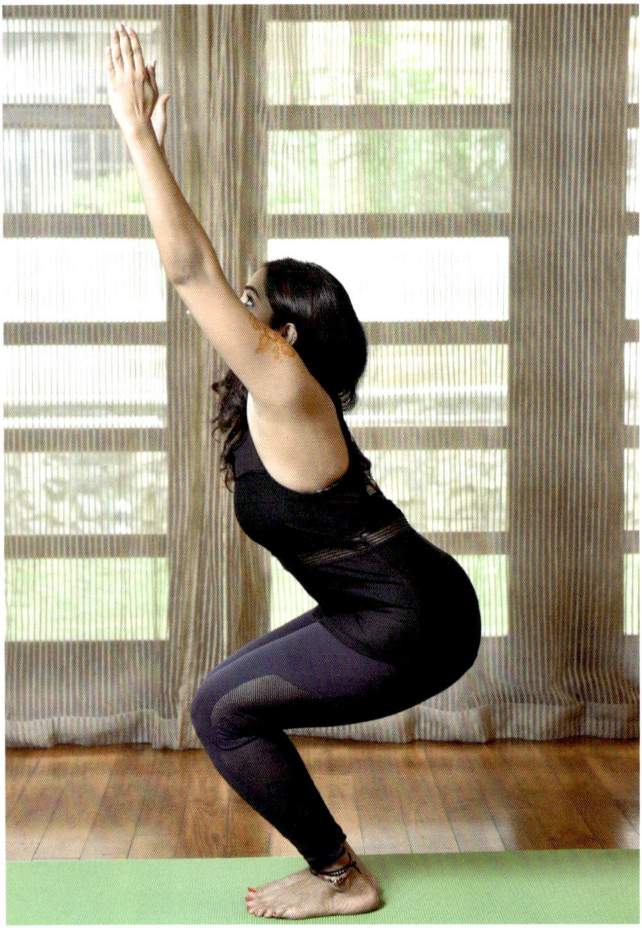

Utkatasana

1. Stand with your feet together. Bend your knees and lower your sit bones downward and backward.
2. Inhale, lift your side and back ribs, and raise your arms up. Keep your elbows straight and press your palms into each other if possible. Gaze upward towards your thumbs
3. Feel the lengthening of the sides of your body from the hips all the way upward to the tips of your fingers, and use the strength of the thighs and hips to hold you in this position.

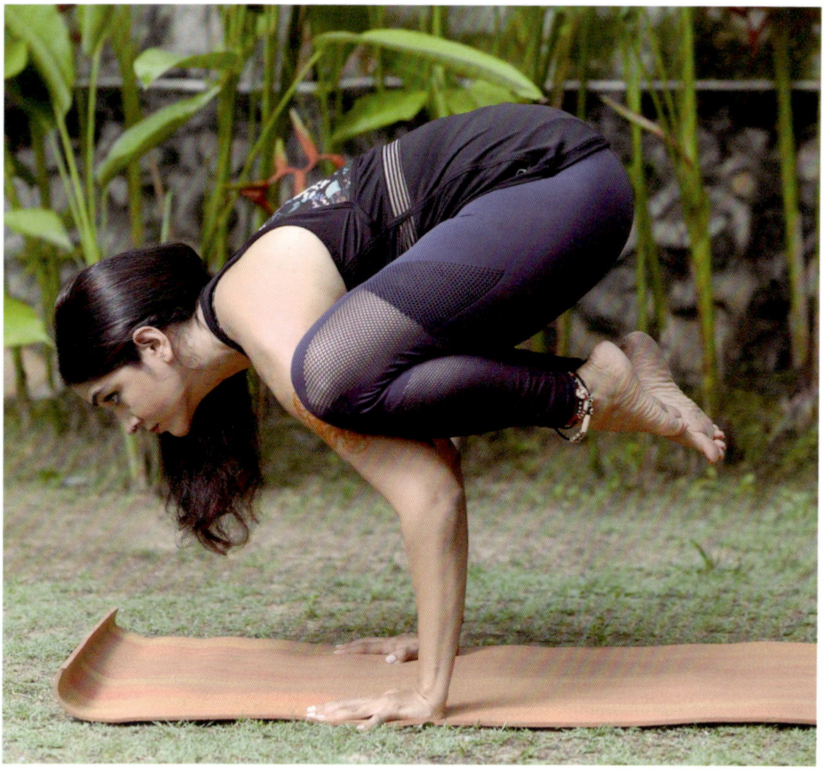

Bakasana

1. Come in to *Malasana* (deep squat, with sit bones near the heels). Place your hands on the floor in front of you.
2. Shift your weight forward from your feet to your palms. Try to take your navel to a point in space directly over your two hands. Then bring your knees to your upper arms, and slowly take your feet off the floor. In the beginning, explore taking one foot at a time off the floor.
3. It is advisable for beginners to place a bolster or a pillow in front of your hands, so that in case you lose balance, as you will be prone to in the beginning, your face will not crash on to the floor.

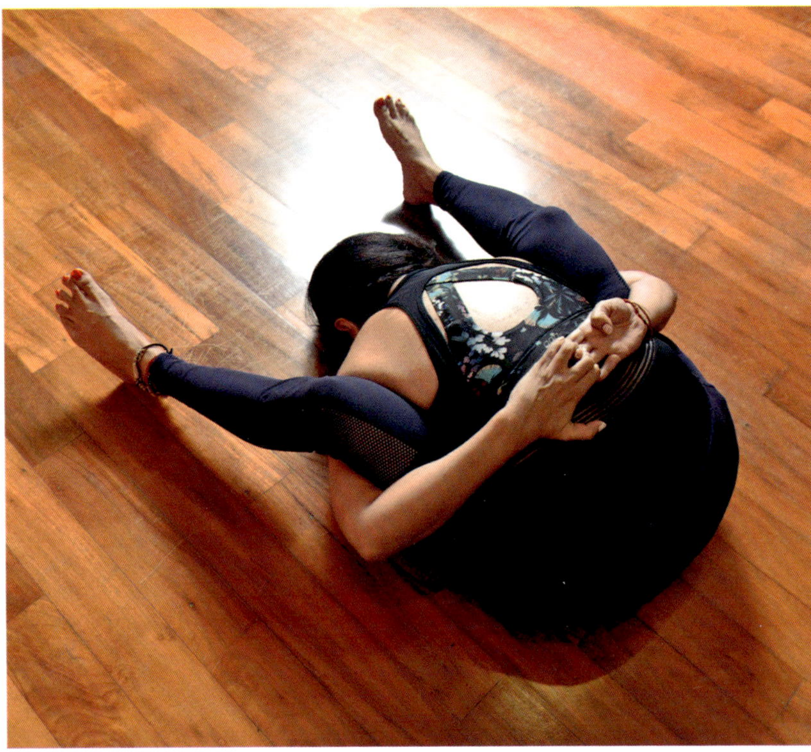

Artistic Pose: *Kurmasana*

Tanu: Thinning, Letting Go

Everything is shown up by being exposed to the light, and whatever is exposed to the light becomes light itself.[1]

—St. Paul

Tanu is the second principle in Manasa yoga. As we begin the pranayama practice, I guide my students to direct their attention to the breath; to be present to its rhythmic flow of inhalation and exhalation. As we strive to retain our attention to the breath, we come face-to-face with distractions that block our ability to experience the moment. These blocks are in the form of anxieties, worries, thoughts of being wronged, justifications, sadness, memories of times gone by, need for vengeance, a conversation we just had etc. Again and again, almost helplessly, the thoughts flow in the same grooves and we remain stuck to a particular story or perspective. This also prevents us from opening our hearts to receive the moment.

1 Eckhart Tolle, *The Power of Now: A Guide to Spiritual Enlightenment* (Vancouver, Canada: Namaste Publishing and Novato, California: New World Library, 1999).

This is also true with any other scenario in life; when we are with our family we worry about deadlines, when we are at work we wonder whether our kids made it to school on time, when we are watching a beautiful sunset we think about booking an Uber and making it to the airport on time to catch our flight! And we live most of our lives in this unconscious manner, never being really present. Thus the relevance and need for *tanu*—thinning, or the ability to consciously let go of whatever is unnecessary to the moment. Otherwise, these stresses act as blocks, and hang over us like dark clouds, colouring our every experience of life, and ultimately rendering us unable to sink into the moment.

Patanjali mentions *tanukaranam* in the second sutra of the second chapter of the *Yoga Sutras*:

Samadhi bhavanaarthah klesha tanukaranarthasca
To cultivate states of samadhi, it is important to thin down (tanukaranam) *afflictions* (kleshas)[2]

Kleshas

So what are *kleshas*? *Kleshas* are the proverbial choppy restless waves, the afflictions that agitate the ocean of our consciousness. In the third verse of the second chapter, Patanjali lists the *kleshas* as *avidya* (ignorance or misapprehension), *asmita* (false identity), *raga* (desire, attachment, passion), *dvesha* (hatred, dislike, enmity) and *abhinivesha* (insecurity, fear of death). We will explore the *kleshas* further in the next chapter.

States of Mind

Sage Vyasa classifies five states of the mind:

Kshipta (state of restlessness)

2 'Manasa Yoga' *Teacher Training Notes.*

Mudha (state of dullness)
Vikshipta (intermittent state between wandering and staying)

But the state of samadhi would arise only in:
Ekagra (state of concentrated absorption)
Niruddha (state of dissolution)

The stretch of yoga is the stretch of the mind from states of kshipta to ekagra, from states of agitation, restlessness and reactivity towards states of calmness, centeredness and one-pointedness.

—Manoj Kaimal

The practice of yoga invites us to shift from being stuck, inflexible and rigid in our thinking to being more open, flexible and accommodative. From releasing the need to cling to beliefs and perception on how life, love, children, people etc., should be, regardless of how much we have staked our life on it, and becoming more open and non-judgmental of the way the universe flows and unfolds in our lives. When we hold on tightly to how things should be, how people should respond, or how situations should turn out, it only leads to suffering, as we become non-accepting of how life unfolds.

From conditional to unconditional, from demand to acceptance, from control to surrender—that is the path of yoga.

All suffering is the result of resistance; the non-acceptance of 'What-IS' in the present moment.

What Does Letting Go Involve?

Letting go calls for us to take a good, long and hard look at ourselves and the state of our lives. It demands that we define what our values are, what we stand for, what we will accept and what we will not. It calls for us to remove the rose-tinted blinkers that we love to wear over our eyes and come face-to-face with the reality of actions and situations, beyond our mind's own stories and beliefs, beyond our desires and limited perceptions—that we are indispensable to our company, that our job will last forever, that our partner will never cheat on us, that situations and people will always remain the same.

It requires us to accept that we have to reassess a person, a situation or a job, that we may have to rewrite the script of our lives. Letting go applies across the board—with regard to a dead-end job, a meaningless relationship, an eating pattern that is slowly but surely killing us, an alcohol addiction that is ruining not just us but the lives of people around us too. The discord and pain that we suffer is our inner self urging us to value ourselves, stand our ground and release whatever takes us away from our inner alignment.

Action and Consequence

The only thing to bear in mind is that every action has a consequence. So when we let go of a certain aspect of our life, we have to be conscious that there will be consequences that follow; that things cannot remain the same. It's part of the deal. A lot of the times, we realize that a certain situation makes us feel bad but because we are so compulsively caught up in it, we are unable to free ourselves, even if it takes us to the point of self-destruction. Many-a-time we hold on to something because we are unable to come to terms with change in the status quo—moving out of a marriage, having to change jobs and move to a different city, a different country, moving out of a (disagreeable) comfort zone, having to face life on our own etc. But release and move forward into the dark expanse of the unknown we must, if we are to break free from the wretchedness and hopelessness that encases our hearts and breaks our spirit.

The ability to self-destruct is dangerously real. There are people who continue to smoke and drink even though they have been diagnosed with cancer, who are unable to change eating patterns (like stopping the consumption of sweets) even in the face of being diagnosed as pre-diabetic, who stay on in dead-end jobs because they cannot endure the process of looking for another, who hold onto relationships though there is no love or respect because it is too hard to think of life in terms of living alone. But it only leads to a slow eroding of self-worth, and ultimately, self-destruction.

Aham Baddha Vimuktasya Aham

I am bound. I want to be free

—the twin aspects of bondage and freedom inspired from the ancient scripture, *Yoga Vasishta*

When we sit in silence and our mind is calm, we should gently ask ourselves, what blocks our joy? The answers will come in clear images or in the form of conversations of situations that we find ourselves in that do not honour us. But we settle because we believe that there is no other way open to us. We lock ourselves in, bind ourselves and, for good measure, throw the keys away as well.

Usually, it is through great pain and intense suffering that we come to the realization that it is we who have locked ourselves in, and have nailed the boards in for good measure. This happens because of our obstinate beliefs about a particular person, job, situation or life, our unwillingness to accept that our beliefs may have been wrong and we may not be on the correct path, our own insecurities and lack of confidence, and our lack of value for ourselves and low self-esteem.

Thus, it is important to keep expanding our worlds, opening our minds, broadening our perspectives. We have to know that there are always options and that only we hold the keys that can unlock the prison doors of suffering that we have shackled ourselves in. We have to take responsibility for the state of our minds and the state of our lives. And only we can do that. We have to unravel the knots ourselves; knot by knot, pattern by pattern, day-by-day, through the empowering process of letting go.

'Unconsciousness creates it; consciousness transmutes it into itself.'[3]

—Eckhart Tolle

The Secret to Letting Go

But even as we intellectually understand the need to let go, how do we let go? Is there a magic wand that we can wave around and swoosh! All is forgotten, all is well! No, it doesn't work that way. In fact, the paradox is that the more our focus is directed on letting something go, the more we are gripped by it, consumed by it almost!

The illustrious yogi Sri Sri Paramahansa Yogananda says,

> *Mental slavery to a sense habit is the result of continued repetition of the specific act that gives birth to a particular habit. By attentively thinking about a certain thing every day, an individual makes that thing a part of his consciousness. When a habit becomes an integral facet of one's thought, it becomes 'second nature'. This 'second nature' is so powerful*

3 Eckhart Tolle, *The Power of Now: A Guide to Spiritual Enlightenment* (Vancouver, Canada: Namaste Publishing and Novato, California: New World Library, 1999).

> *it convinces one that he can never get rid of his own 'nature', even if in exchange he were to receive a whole world of superior satisfaction.*[4]

So what is the answer? The answer is to **SHIFT OUR FOCUS**!

For that we need to be aware that as human beings, we are all endowed with the powerful capacity of CHOICE. This again is a term we are unfamiliar with as most of the time we just function helplessly on the likes and dislikes of the mind. But as we become seasoned yoga practitioners, as we align more and more to our core, we become more conscious of the vagaries of the mind and don't feel so deeply identified with it. We are able to 'see' the anger, the depression, the rage, the obsessions and compulsions, and the gripping attachment without always lashing out and reacting to it.

We may not all be able to physically let go or walk away from situations, but with consistent practice we can all make the mental shift to consciously direct our attention to areas of our lives that work, that bring us meaning and joy and fulfill us. For some of us our work may be going well, for some others with financial problems, their family lives may be the source of their satisfaction, and for yet some others it may be the support of long-term friendships. We all have positive areas in our lives, areas that work, that come easily. The key is to be aware of them (as opposed to always being lost in complaining and dissatisfaction), consciously bring our attention to them, focus on them and allow them to expand.

4 Paramahansa Yogananda, *God Talks With Arjuna: The Bhagavad Gita* (Kolkata: Yagoda Satsanga Society of India, 2011).

Negativity Bias

This is conscious work as the 'negativity bias' runs deep in all of us. Negativity bias is an accepted human phenomenon where *negative* experiences tend to exert a greater psychological impact on us than positive experiences of the same magnitude. Scientists say that it is an evolutionary adaptation that we react to bad or dangerous things more quickly and persistently than to good things. It suggests that our minds are hardwired to be naturally skewed towards negativity, as a result of which we tend to remember more insults than praise—the one person who didn't congratulate us though a 100 other people did, the one girl who was mean to us in school more than 20 years ago though we aren't in contact with that person now. This can have a devastating effect on our emotions and our lives, as it gets integrated into our belief systems and we just live and act out of it.

We have to develop the capacity to 'see' the negative workings of the mind, the same patterns of judgment—this is bad, he is evil, she is conniving, money is the root of evil. We may have self-defeating thoughts—I am never going to be successful, I don't have what it takes to be wealthy, I am fated to be disappointed in love. We may even develop a victim mentality—he did this to me, I am unsuccessful today because my parents never loved me, if I were more beautiful I would be happier ... the list goes on. Only when we become conscious of the working of the mind can we take back our power to shift our perspective and break the loop of thought, think differently and thus, bring about a change in the state of our minds and, eventually, our lives.

As is our inner world so is our outer world. All the work is in our hearts—to keep it open in the face of resistance, heartbreak and grief, and to be able to receive life as it unfolds. That is the *tapas* (intense effort), that is the journey, that is the yoga!

Practice

1. What patterns block your happiness?
2. What do you find most hard to let go of, though you know it is not good for you?
3. What is it you fear the most if you let go of that pattern?
4. What are you compromising by holding on to the situation? Is it your dignity? Your self-respect? Your sanity? Your lifestyle?

Asanas: Bound Asanas

In life, we bind ourselves consciously or unconsciously through our thoughts and actions. Ultimately, in the yearning for freedom and liberation, we have to unlock and release ourselves. We embody that in our asana practice with a bound sequence.

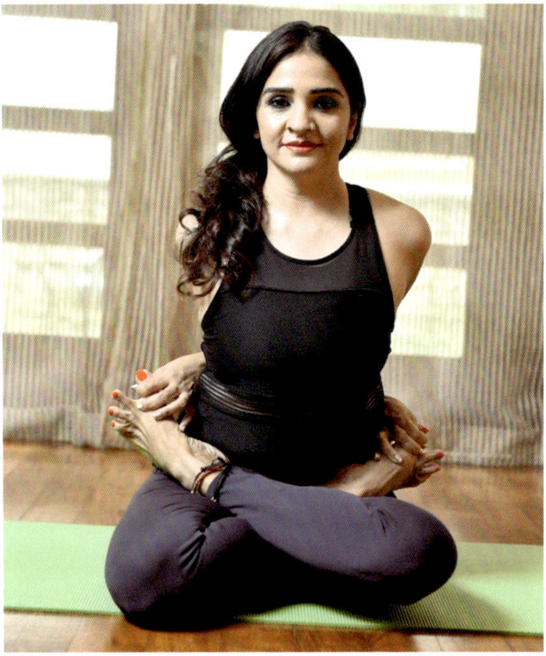

Baddha Padmasana: Bound Lotus

1. Sit with your legs stretched out in front of you.
2. Externally rotate your right hip, bend your right leg, catch hold of your right foot with both hands and carefully bring the heel of your right foot to the left hip crease.
3. Very carefully, do the same with your left foot. Since a sideways pulling of the shin is possible here (which can potentially cause an injury), it is advisable to learn the lotus asana under the supervision of an experienced teacher.

For the bound position, it is important to try and get both heels as close to your hip as possible. This results in a closely bound lotus and allows you to open your shoulders and take your arms behind your torso to hold your toes. First, take one arm behind your body and hold your big toe, then lean towards the other side to hold the other big toe.

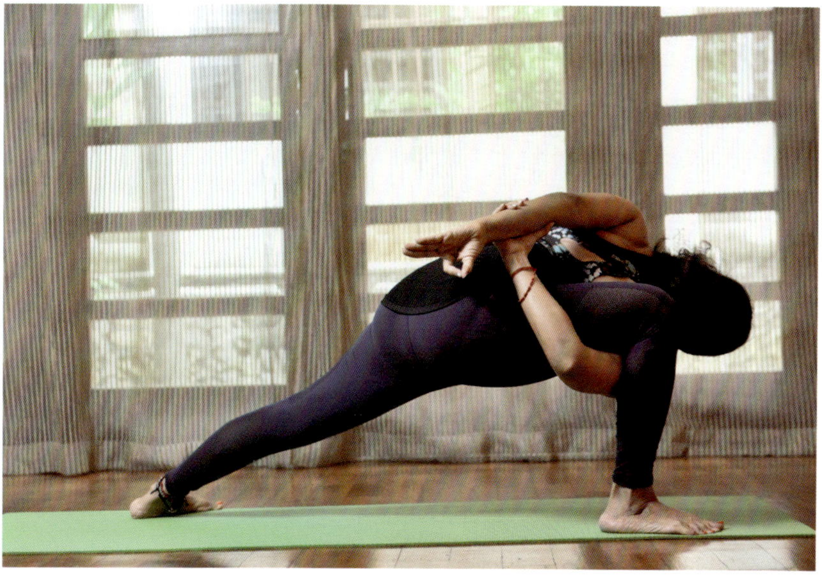

Baddha Parsvakonasana: Bound Lateral Angle Pose

1. Keep your feet wide apart. Turn your right leg out to the right. Bend your right knee until your knee is directly over your right heel. Slide your left foot away as much as needed so that you can lower your right buttock down to be in line with your right knee. Lean to the right and place your right palm on the floor besides your right foot. Take your left arm over your ear and lengthen the side body. This is *parsvakonasana* or the lateral angle position.
2. From here, as you exhale, lower your right shoulder below your right thigh, internally rotate your right shoulder, bend your right elbow and reach towards your right outer thigh/ hip with your right hand.
3. Now externally rotate your left shoulder and take your left arm back and down. Catch your left wrist with your right hand if possible. Otherwise use a strap and hold one side of the strap in each hand

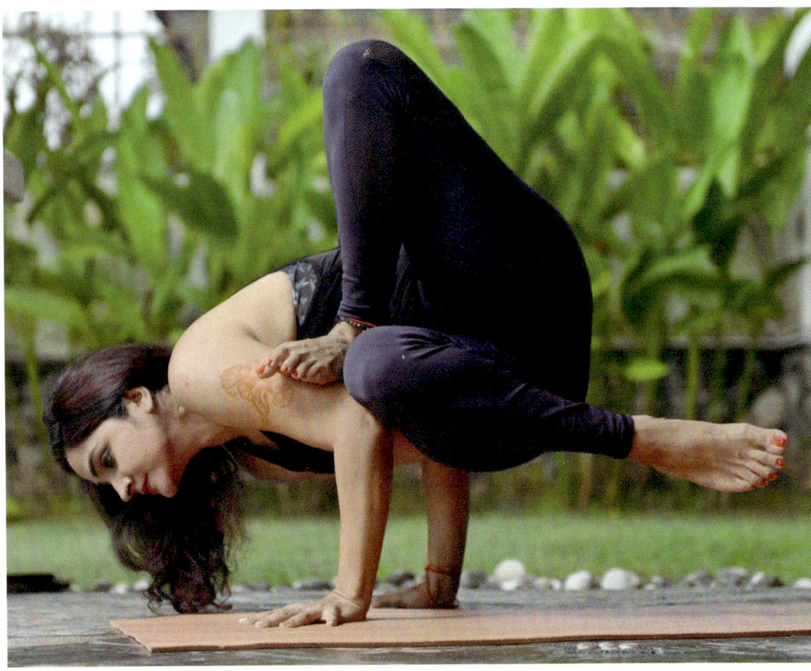

Artistic Pose: *Parivritta Galavasana*

Suffering Through the Lens of *Kleshas*

Vivekakhyatiraviplava hanopayah

Freedom from suffering can only be realized through 'viveka', discriminatory wisdom.[1]

—Patanjali's *Yoga Sutras*, chapter 2, sutra 26

The area of relationships has a profound emotional effect on our lives, and we usually have little or no support to cope with the devastation when it ends. I have also received numerous messages, and had many conversations with friends having relationship struggles or going through divorce, and have discussed the baggage of trauma that comes with it. The wisdom of the sutras can be applied to all situations in life where we suffer.

A relationship is one area where we invest all our emotions. But sometimes, choices are made for us. People decide to leave and close doors on us. It has the power to scar us, leaving the

1 'Manasa Yoga' *Teacher Training Notes.*

wounds raw and bleeding for a lifetime. All this can leave us bitter and resentful, souring our very experience of life. It can result in severe psychological trauma, leading to anxiety, chronic depression, or post-traumatic stress disorder.

So it is important, for our own sakes, to feel acceptance, make peace with the situation, and move forward with our lives. And what enables us to do that is, understanding. In the second chapter of the *Yoga Sutras*, Patanjali lists five *kleshas*, or afflictions. When I first heard of them, they all came together and made perfect sense, like pieces of a puzzle. Each of them spoke to me like old friends bringing me greater clarity, having come face to face with them at one point or another through different life experiences

Avidya is considered the breeding-ground of all other *kleshas*, as the lack of true knowledge is the source of all pain, whether dormant or active. *Asmita* refers to egoism that develops as a result of the ignorance of the true self.

Raga

Raga or deep attachment is touted as one of the afflictions or *kleshas* that must be overcome for clear seeing. This is because excessive attachment literally makes us blind and additionally, comes with a whole family of other related emotions like intense cravings, compulsions, obsessions, unreasonableness, demands, desire for control, and extreme mood swings and behaviours.

It all begins with an innocuous liking. For example, when we come across a person, an object or a pattern that brings us pleasure. Consciously or unconsciously, our actions are inspired around keeping those pleasure circuits going. So we hang around the person, walk around with our phones in our hands and check our WhatsApp group every few minutes! All is well in our world. But unbeknown to us, it slowly turns into an insidious pattern, creating addictive neural networks and patterns that holds us in its obsessive-compulsive grip. *Raga* could also develop with regard to a position we hold dear, say a corporate title, or an eating, drinking or lifestyle pattern that has a hold on us, or it could even develop because of social media.

Dvesha

If we possess the object of our attachment for even a while, it gives us happiness, but on the flip side, if we lose our object of happiness or if the object does not respond the way we would like it to, then it plunges us into deep suffering!

So when the relationship ends, what we come face-to-face with is not *raga* (though it began with that) but its twin, *dvesha*. The sadness, anger, disbelief, bitterness, and the rage that *dvesha* causes can be overwhelming. This is because, over a period of time, we have identified ourselves so closely with another person at the cost of our own selves, and intertwined our lives with theirs, that when the breakup happens, it shocks us to our very core.

A lot of breakups around the world have led to violent and tragic consequences. These are the manifestations of thwarted attachment. People have even been driven to kill when the object of their attachment forsakes them. Which is why it is all the more important that we come into an understanding and accept the situation. If we watch the movement of the mind carefully, we can see that these twin principles of *raga* and *dvesha* can be applied to any life situation. Anything that we have a deep attachment to has the potential to transform into *dvesha* if we are unconscious about it. In yoga class too we can have a *raga* and become fixated on certain kinds of classes, or specific end points in an asana—balance in handstand, palms flat in *uttanasana* (the standing forward fold)—and then move into *dvesha* and get disheartened and frustrated if that doesn't happen. In the process, we lose out on the whole joy of the 'process' of asana.

Raga and *dvesha* can be applied to people's deep identification with their jobs and positions too. Recently, I heard of a friend's husband who went into deep depression and alcoholism after being laid off at the age of fifty-four from a company he had been with since he was twenty-two. It is because our identification with our jobs is so complete that when we lose it, it is like the carpet being pulled out from beneath our feet. We cannot come to terms with it and imagine a life without it. Disregarding the obvious addictions of alcohol or tobacco, a lot of people today are in the grip of addiction to their diet and lifestyle patterns. I do not say this without any basis. Worldwide, obesity is considered an epidemic of growing proportions. This is again the reflection of our inability to make the necessary changes to our diet and lifestyle because of our deep attachment to food and the dislike of the discomfort that goes along with changing our food habits and lifestyle patterns. India, in particular, has the dubious distinction of being known as the 'Diabetic Capital of the World!' with more than 50 million people diagnosed with Type 2 diabetes. Lifestyle modifications, which include changes in diet and exercise patterns, are recognized and accepted worldwide as the keys to controlling it.

Avidya

Avidya, the lack of knowledge or misapprehension, is considered the breeding ground of all other *kleshas*. We have to take responsibility for the state of our lives and emotions. We have to realize that it is our own lack of understanding or knowledge about the person or the situation, our misplaced beliefs about our relationship or position in the company, or the lack of consciousness of our eating and lifestyle patterns that have contributed to our suffering. Our deep attachment and dependence is assiduously cultivated, unconsciously, over time, through our inability to accept the situation and make changes—to alter our lifestyle and food habits or risk being diagnosed as diabetic; that our journey with our previous company is over and we have to open our minds and be willing to make changes like move to another country, learn a new set of skills, another language etc. to get another job; that maybe we have to give up the comfort of a luxurious lifestyle to be authentic to ourselves. Whatever may be the situation, our resistance to what IS, results in our pain.

In chapter 2, sutra 5, Patanjali goes on to elaborate on the various *avidya*s or misapprehensions that arise: as we mistake *anitya* for *nitya*, the impermanent for the permanent; anatma for atma, the non-self for the self; and *asuchi* for *suchi*, the impure for the pure.

Of them, the concept of impermanence, *anitya*, invited me to explore deeper into the human psyche and its need for permanence. As human beings, we believe and get lulled into a false sense of complacency that all things will always be the same, although nature is always showing us things to the contrary. Everything in nature speaks of impermanence. A seed is planted, it sprouts, the tree grows and blossoms and it dies. It is the same with human beings and animals—they all go through a cycle of birth, growth, maturity, decay and death. Similarly, if we explore the breath—an inhalation is born, it expands to its maximum potential and then it dies as the exhalation is born. When our children grow up and leave the nest to study, and eventually have families of their own, there is an altering in the relationship that is inevitable. All experiences have a beginning and an end. Things, people, relationships, jobs are shifting all the time. There is no permanence, and yet we constantly seek it, and in our inability to accept it, suffer deeply for it.

Abhinivesha

Abhinivesha is traditionally defined as the fear of death that develops as a result of our deep attachment to life. Contemplation on the concept of 'death' opened up a whole new dimension to life. I realised that 'death' did not have to be limited to just the physical body. We come face-to-face with death more often than we realize. There is death in the context of relationships as the dynamics of a relationship are always fluid: between parents and children, friends, lovers, business partners, and siblings. There is a difference in the need and dependence a baby has for its mother, and that of a boy leaving for college. The closeness between siblings when they were all young and stayed in the same house will be different as they spread their wings and nest in different parts of the world. In the current economic scenario, job security is a thing of the past, especially in the corporate arena. So there is death in the context of a loss of the job or change in position. As my expatriate students pack their houses and lifestyles as they move from Malaysia to other countries, there is *abhinivesha* there too. Again, there is the death of hopes, dreams, beliefs, and attitudes as life happens and our minds open, sometimes naturally and sometimes forcefully, to a different perspective. *Abhinivesha* lurks in the fringes of our lives, but ever so often it surges to the forefront, overwhelming us with anxieties, insecurities, feelings of loss of control of our emotions and moods as we struggle to come to terms with the twists and turns that life seems to delight in throwing at us.

Self-Love and Respect

When we love and respect ourselves, all other relationships fall into place.

In the name of love, we actually give our power away. The deeper the attachment and the more bound we are, the more of ourselves we give away. Many a time, in order to desperately hold on to a relationship, a job or even a food or an alcohol pattern, we compromise our values, our self-respect and we become a far cry from the person we were meant to be.

Another's action or inaction has the power to deeply affect us—our emotions, our moods, our state of mind and ultimately, our lives. We constantly seek validity and approval from others and from the state of our relationships. We train ourselves in this manner to look outside of ourselves. As long as someone is giving us their undivided attention, life is hunky-dory, but when their attention goes away, then we struggle to make sense of our lives. We have no idea about the person we have turned out to be. What is important to us? What is our path?

If the bonds are deep, then it may take a while to release them. But what is most important is the conscious desire to release them. And that only comes from a place of wisdom and clarity, from *viveka*. The most empowering aspect of yoga is that it enhances our awareness and sensitivity to ourselves, our thoughts, our actions, our moods, the state of our minds and lives. As our ability to continuously watch ourselves deepens, we gain wisdom and clarity. There is less and less confusion about our path. We see the futility of it all—the emptiness in words, the actions that reflect a lack of value and respect, our blind beliefs, our deep attachment, the triggers and our reactivity. And we see our light slowly but surely growing dimmer and dimmer, smothered below layers of pain, depression, anxiety, mood swings, reactivity, rage and a general lack of interest in life itself! Again, when we allow an eating or a drinking pattern to take over our lives, our bodies and minds do not reflect the value we have for ourselves. We were all born to achieve our highest potential—physically, mentally and emotionally. Yet, in the grip of unhealthy eating and drinking patterns, we let it all slip by the wayside.

It is only the grace of wisdom, with its sharp sword of discernment, that can sever the deep bonds of attachment; beyond the desperate need that makes us want to cling and hold on, and remain in places where we are not honoured, or worse, which take us steadily downhill.

Lessons From the Contrast

We come to the realization that the highest state is to be able to see the learning and evolve. When things don't turn out the way we expected, when we can get past the sadness and the grief, what shines through like a glowing beacon, is the learning that we received through the contrast. It is through the contrast that we gain sharp clarity about ourselves. What exactly do we want in a relationship or a person or a job? How do we want to be treated? What do we stand for? What are our values? What are we willing to live with?

When we experience being treated without value, then we connect deeply, almost instinctively, to our love and respect for ourselves. The process of owning our power and self-respect demands a release of old patterns of suffering and embracing new ways of thinking and living that enhances self-love and respect. So ironically, the very act of releasing is an act of empowerment, a step towards wholeness.

The greatest act of self-love is to consciously release people and situations that afflict us and, in the process, allow our inherent light to shine resplendent.

The same holds good for other experiences as well. If we were in a job situation with a boss from hell, then it connects us to what is important in our lives, i.e., to be treated with respect and value. If we suffer from ill-health, we appreciate the value of good health and we take steps to change patterns and improve our health. If we are overweight and don't possess the svelte figure that we dreamed of, we begin to appreciate the importance of our diet and exercise patterns. If we suffer mentally from agitation, frustration and reactivity, then we yearn for peace, which in turn would cause us to seek out a yoga class or a meditation course.

So, in all ways, we are being refined through our life experiences and directed to live from our authentic aligned state.

And as we consciously release negative patterns and energies from our lives, our light shines bright and magically connects us to deep dormant reserves of positive energy that attract similar persons and situations that enable us to evolve into our highest possibilities, our greatest selves. So bless the contrast.

I was recently in conversation with a friend who was struggling to come to terms with the fact that his wife had decided to end their marriage, despite his best efforts to reconcile and hold on. Faith and surrender were the only words I could offer faith in the greater universal plan, and our surrender to it despite our inability to understand its workings at this point of time in our lives. *Ishwara pranidhana.* Surrendering to a higher force, a recognition that we are not the ultimate masters of our fate allows us to assimilate change in a way that empowers us and promotes our continuous evolvement, and the flow of our consciousness into auspicious (*kalyana*) states of acceptance, appreciation and gratitude.

We must walk in the expanded awareness that everything is part of the larger tapestry of life. It is only in hindsight, when we look back, that we will see the synchronicity of it all, that the dots will connect. We must stop our minds from judging and labeling every single experience in our lives as good or bad because the truth is that, with our limited perspective, we really don't know. At that point it may seem like a failure, but later when we look back we will realize that we were being directed towards our greater destiny.

As Steve Jobs said in his commencement address at Stanford University in 2005:

> *You can't connect the dots looking forward; you can only connect them looking backwards. So you have to trust that the dots will somehow connect in your future. You have to trust in something—your gut, destiny, life, karma, whatever. This approach has never let me down, and has made all the difference in my life.*

This is one of my favorite stories, a Chinese parable, and it offers me a lot of comfort when I come across a situation that my mind hastens to judge (as it loves to) as shattering, difficult, end-of-the-world etc. It is a reminder that what can often be seen as a misfortune can turn into a very good thing.

The Old Man and His Horse

> *Once there was an old man who lived in a tiny village. Although poor, he was envied by all, for he owned a beautiful white horse.*

Even the king coveted his treasure. People offered fabulous prices for the steed, but the old man always refused. 'This horse is not a horse to me,' he would tell them. 'He is a friend, not a possession. How could you sell a friend?' The man was poor and the temptation was great. But he never sold the horse.

One morning he found that the horse was not in his stable. The entire village came to see him. 'You old fool,' they scoffed, 'we told you that someone would steal your horse. It would have been better to have sold him. You could have gotten whatever price you wanted. Now the horse is gone and you've been cursed with misfortune.' The old man responded, 'Don't speak too quickly. Say only that the horse is not in the stable. That is all we know; the rest is judgment. If I've been cursed or not, how can you know? How can you judge?' The people contested, 'Don't make us out to be fools! We may not be philosophers, but great philosophy is not needed. The simple fact that your horse is gone is a curse.' The old man spoke again. 'All I know is that the stable is empty, and the horse is gone. The rest I don't know. Whether it be a curse or a blessing, I can't say. All we can see is a fragment. Who can say what will come next?'

After fifteen days, the horse returned. He hadn't been stolen; he had run away into the forest. Not only had he returned, he had brought a dozen wild horses with him. Once again, the village people gathered around the woodcutter and spoke. 'Old man, you were right and we were wrong. What we thought was a curse was a blessing. Please forgive us.' The man responded, 'Once again, you go too far. Say only that the horse is back. State only that a dozen horses returned with him, but don't judge. How do you know if this is a blessing or not? You see only a fragment. Unless you know the whole story, how can you judge? You read only one page of a book. Can you judge the whole book? You read only one word of one phrase. Can you understand the entire phrase? Life is so vast, yet you judge all of life with one page or one word.'

The old man had a son, an only son. The young man began to break the wild horses. After a few days, he fell from one of the horses and broke both legs. Once again the villagers gathered around the old man and cast their judgment. 'You were right,' they said. 'You proved you were right. The dozen horses were not a blessing. They were a curse. Your only son has broken both his legs, and now in your old age you have no one to help you.' The old man spoke again. 'You people are obsessed with judging. Don't go so far. Say only that my son broke his legs. Who knows if it is a blessing or a curse? No one knows. We only have a fragment. Life comes in fragments.'

It so happened that a few weeks later the country engaged in war against a neighboring country. All the young men of the village were required to join the army. Only the son of the old man was excluded, because he was injured. Once again the people gathered around the old man, crying and screaming because their sons had been taken. There was little chance that they would return. The enemy was strong, and the war would be a losing struggle. They would never see their sons again. 'You were right, old man,' they wept. 'God knows you were right. This proves it. Your son's accident was a blessing. His legs may be broken, but at least he is with you. Our sons are gone forever.' The old man spoke again. 'It is impossible to talk with you. You always draw conclusions. No one knows. Say only this. Your sons had to go to war, and mine did not. No one knows if it is a blessing or a curse. No one is wise enough to know. Only God knows.'[2]

2 Therese J. Borchard, The Old Man and His Horse. World of Psychology (blog), PsychCentral, 22 July, 2010, https://psychcentral.com/blog/the-old-man-and-his-horse/

Life can only be understood backwards, but it must be lived forwards. So we must proceed with courage towards new doors that open for us, into the magic that the universe spins for us, holding up mirrors and showing us hitherto hidden parts of ourselves in roles that we have only dreamt of, the stuff dreams are made of!

'Forgiveness is so important. We have all done those things for which we condemn others. We must forgive others'.[3]

—Dr Brian Weiss

Practice

1. Identify your support system: a friend or family member who can talk you through your pain and anguish.
2. Create a daily ritual of writing in a journal. Writing a journal is a powerful tool that helps you get in touch with yourself and express your pent-up tormented emotions. It lends you great insights into yourself and the workings of the relationship as well as aspects of the relationship that you may have been formerly blind to.
3. Make peace with the unknown. Be willing to explore life and push the boundaries. Have faith in a larger plan that will unfold in its own time. You will be truly amazed at the guidance and support that will come into your life when you most need it.
4. Space and time, in that particular order, are the best healers.

Asana: Twists

The journey of life constantly throws twists and turns along the way. So becoming adept at dealing with the twists on the mat allows us to flow with the challenges and surprises of life.

---

3 Brian Weiss, *Only Love is Real: A Story of Soulmates Reunited* (New York: Warner Books Inc., 2000).

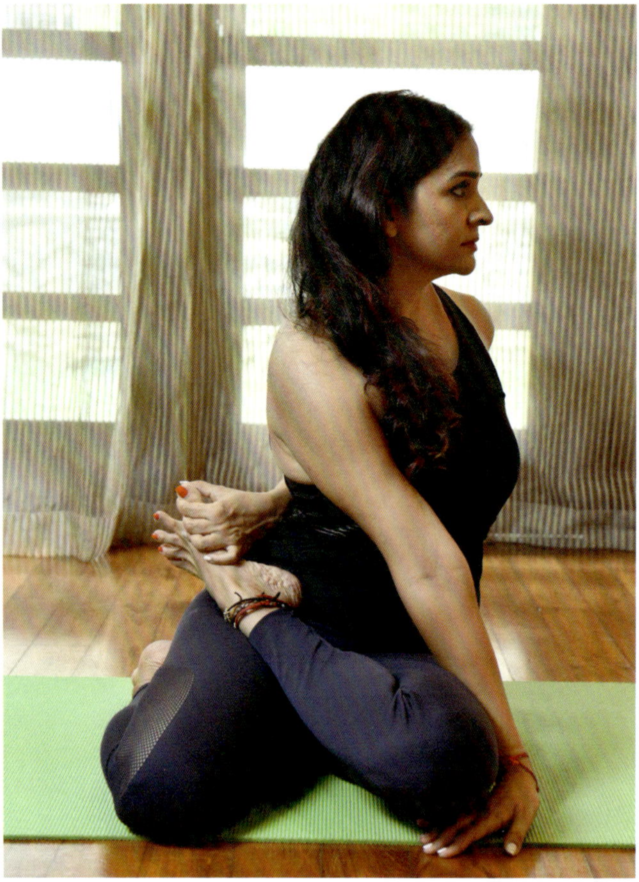

Bharadwajasana

1. Sit on the floor with your legs straight in front. Bend your left leg back, so that your left foot is beside your left buttock. Now externally rotate your right hip and bring your right foot on to your left thigh, close to the left hip crease.
2. Take your right arm back, and bind your right foot with your right hand. If not, use a strap to be looped around the foot and bind the loop.
3. Place your left palm under your right knee, and twist strongly to the right. Look to the side.
4. Stay for 5–10 breaths and repeat on the other side.

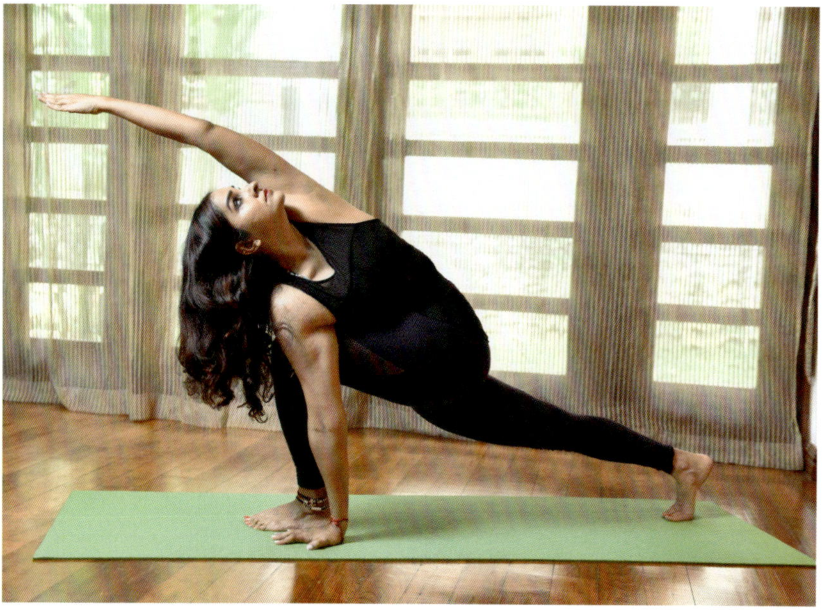

Parivrtta Parsvakonasana: Rotated Lateral Angle

1. Stand with your feet at hip-width. Keep your hands on your hips, with your fingertips facing each other. Inhale and take a step back with your left foot, while still maintaining the pelvis square and keeping your hands on your hips.
2. Exhale as you bend your right knee, until your knee is over your heel, and your right buttock is in line with your right knee. The back of your left heel can be lifted off the floor.
3. Exhale again, as you twist and take your left upper arm across and down the outside of your right thigh. If your armpit touches your outer knee, then lower your left hand to the floor, twist your ribs towards the ceiling and take your right arm overhead.
4. Beginners can just bring their palms into a namaste across the knee and keep the twist going towards the right.
5. Hold for 5–8 breaths and repeat on the other side.

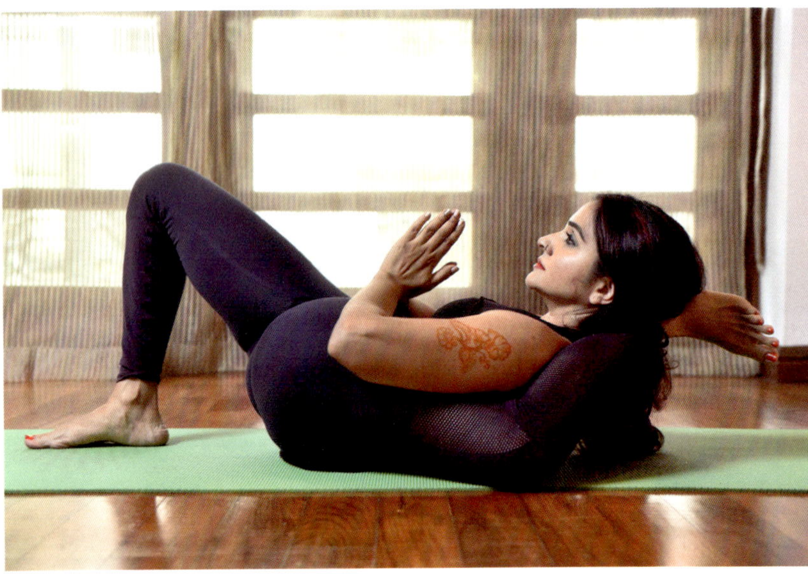

Artistic Pose: *Kashyapasana*

Meeting Suffering

Out of suffering have emerged the strongest souls; the most massive characters are seared with scars.[1]

—Khalil Gibran

Why does my book delve so much into suffering? Because pain and suffering are catalysts that jolt us out of our comfort zones; to search, to seek, to understand, to expand. It comes down to perspective. When things fall apart, when we lose a job, a relationship ends, or we have health problems, our whole perspective of life shifts. Till then we are ruled by the senses, and the mind is outward bound, constantly seeking gratification through acquiring and aggrandizing. Running into a wall is a clarion call that invites us to explore our inner worlds and take a good hard look at the dominant patterns that rule our minds.

We have to push through the borders of our comfort zones, bolster our courage and come face-to-face with our insecurities

1 Khalil Gibran, *The Broken Wings* (First Rate Publishers, 2015).

and our deepest fears. We have to be able to see clearly behind the masks of artifice and make-believe—the stories, imagination, jealousy, envy, hatred, attachments, need for control, viciousness—and work through it, in order to be able to connect and expand into our light, into our renewed stronger selves. Only when our minds can shift perspective, release trauma and be in acceptance mode, can we receive life with all its secrets and mysteries. As long as we remain enmeshed in the toxicity of negativity we can never connect to our inner selves and express our light.

'Until we have met the monsters in ourselves, we keep trying to slay them in the outer world. And we find that we cannot. For all darkness in the world stems from darkness in the heart. And it is there that we must do our work.'[2]

—Marianne Williamson

Sarvam Dukham

One of the fruits on the path of yoga is clarity of mind, which brings with it as grace, a release from suffering. Patanjali, in chapter 2, sutra 15 of the *Yoga Sutras*, classifies *dukha* as *tapa dukha, parinama dukha* and *samskara dukha*.

Tapa dukha is the direct experience of pain. A pain in the knee, or a punch in the stomach are all direct experiences of pain. And it's the same with the mind. We often experience intense pain on account of anger, jealousy, hatred etc. So all of us, if we have a body, if we have a mind, are already acquainted with this *dukha* very well.

Parinama dukha is suffering on account of insecurity. If we look at our lives, we perhaps have a job, some savings in the bank,

2 Marianne Williamson, *Everyday Grace: Having Hope, Finding Forgiveness, and Making Miracles* (New York: Bantam Books, 2006).

a house, a partner etc. However, things change all the time, and we can't be secure about anything. We desperately try to build some sense of security in our lives by building our savings, eating multi-vitamins, doing some asana practice etc., but on some level we know that all these things are very dicey. We try to get some emotional stability by getting a stable partner, but we are very quick to doubt and worry because we know deep down that this current stability is also really dicey. The same goes with our jobs. We may have a great job today but beneath that is the insecurity that it could all be gone tomorrow. It's perhaps an intuitive knowledge that though 'now' is good, it needn't be 'forever'. And then we cling. And this act of clinging, where we want to prevent change from happening, is suffering, *parinama dukha*.

Samskara dukha is suffering on account of daily maintenance. In a simple sense, when we wake up every day, there is work: the body has to be taken to the bathroom, the teeth have to be brushed, the body has to be given a shower, fed, cleaned etc. We have built-in mental patterns or *samskaras*. So perhaps, for the mornings, you have built up patterns for how a good morning should be. You should get your coffee or tea at a certain temperature, of a certain brand etc. It was nice in the beginning, but then it becomes a demand. Every morning, these *samskara*s will ask: Where is my coffee? Is the temperature exact? And we will keep on changing it until we get that exact thing, only then will we be happy. It is the same with other routines of our life too. We will check our phone for messages, surf the internet, read the papers, or watch some TV. When we get into our car, music has to be there immediately, otherwise again that *samskara* will demand music, music, music!

All these collective irritations are suffering. They are continuous demands. We have to spend our whole life keeping these patterns entertained and satisfied all the time as they are constantly craving satisfaction. This is, in a simple way, *samskara dukha*.

Through these three teachings, Patanjali tells us that we are suffering, in one way or the other. If you don't want to take Patanjali's word for it, perhaps you might have noticed that when something bad happens to someone, people tell them in a very philosophical tone that 'It's life'.

That's exactly what Patanjali says too. Life is *dukha*.

There is nothing that is not painful: *'sarvam eva dukha mayam'*.

What is the Cause of Suffering?

'Drastr drsyayoho samyogo heya hetuh'

The cause of suffering is when the seer becomes one with the seen (samyoga) *and forgets one's true nature.*[3]

—Patanjali's *Yoga Sutras*, chapter 2, sutra 17

Forgetfulness of one's self as separate—from one's role as father, mother, sister, brother, husband, wife, employer, employee etc., is the main cause of suffering. The seer becomes completely identified with the objects—the car, the job, the watch, the house, the pet, the body, the girlfriend, lover etc. It thinks 'this is me'! The deeper the identification, the more intense the suffering.

The Seamlessness of Mind and Body

In Hatha yoga, we understand that the body is profoundly affected when we experience mental trauma. It does not remain isolated from the happenings of the mind. It tenses in uncertainty, braces in threat, freezes in shock and collapses in hopelessness. This wisdom of the inherent non-divisiveness

3 'Manasa Yoga' *Teacher Traning Notes.*

of body and mind forms the psychological, physiological and spiritual underpinning of yoga.

Recent revolutionary developments in neuroscience have established strong supporting evidence of the intricate two-way communication between mind and body. By identifying complex 'neuro-peptide messengers', researchers like Dr Candace Pert have discovered many pathways by which mind and body mutually communicate. Dr Pert, an American neuroscientist and pharmacologist who discovered the opiate receptor, the cellular binding site for endorphins in the brain, explained that emotions and feelings are not limited only to the brain.

A conscious emotion or feeling occurs when a peptide molecule binds with its receptor. Originally, it was thought that receptors are found only in the brain, but later it was discovered that receptors are found everywhere in the body. Thus, the mind, in its capacity of experiencing, is not just a phenomenon of the brain, but a phenomenon of the whole body. When we say 'gut feeling', it is in fact true. We can feel in our stomachs. So the mind exists everywhere in the body. Thus, via the different asanas, we liberate the mind by freeing ourselves from the ghosts of past trauma, and preventing the breeding of new ones, which, in turn, prevents future suffering. As Patanjali says, '*heyam duhkham anagatham*'—pain that has not yet come is avoidable.

Generally, when the mind's agitator is gone, it returns to a state of apparent normalcy. So though we might think that the erstwhile body's response might have normalized, it actually does not. The body still holds on to many of the characteristics it assumed when the mind was in trauma. So even if we think we are okay, our mind and intellect are still being troubled by traumatic incidents of the past, as the body is still remembering and holding on to the patterns it took upon itself then. Hatha yoga practitioners understand that without accessing the body and mind together as a unit, we will not be able to deeply understand or heal trauma. And the asanas, which seemingly focus on different parts of the body, focus not only on the musculoskeletal stretching of a specific part of the body, but also on releasing traumatic energy/ mind patterns which are held frozen in those areas.

Receive Life

The word 'receive' is such a beautiful word. It implies an invitation to the unfolding of life—a lack of expectation, a lack of demand, a lack of judgment, a lack of condition and an acceptance of life as 'IS'. Most of our pain and suffering in life stems from an inability to accept life as it shows up. We have our own expectations and conditions as to how situations should turn out and how people should behave, but life doesn't always respond the way we would like it to. As we connect to our capacity to receive life, our consciousness flows in a more stable manner.

The Breath

And it begins in yoga class as we receive the breath. As we sit in awareness of the breath, we draw our attention to our inherent capacity to receive as the breath flows towards us. The more we connect to this capacity to receive, the more it deepens and permeates into other aspects of our lives as well. It allows us to slowly release judgment, expectations, conditions, and be more in acceptance of the events and situations we find ourselves in, all of which translates into less suffering!

Mat Practice is Life Practice

Asana practice is a great place to connect and work through life. As we come into awareness of our patterns, we relax on judgments and conditions of 'getting it or not getting it'. We learn not to set the bar on end points or based on other people's bodies, but to connect to every moment of every movement. To find joy in unraveling the process of the asana and pleasure in the fluidity and grace of our bodies, the stretch of the hamstrings, the resistance of the adductors, the lengthening of the spine, the pressure on our palms, the steadiness of the body, the evenness of our breaths, the tranquility of our minds, as the asana reveals itself to us.

And, as we learn to stay with both—the motivation to move deeper into possibility of movement, but at the same time, instead of fighting harshly with resistance, trying to accommodate it, face it with love and compassion—we eventually elicit a release. So in the body, area by area, we create relaxation and strength which spills over into the psyche, giving us an overall sense of release. Physiologically, the sustained stretch will eventually lead to a relaxation response (reciprocal inhibition principle) in the opposing muscles, provided we were not forcing our position. If we are to grit through pain, then the effect will be contrary, creating excitatory, unsettling patterns, where we end up increasing the conflicts within, between different parts of our own nervous system.

With consistent attunement, these attitudes of accommodation, compassion and kindness to our bodies slowly become ingrained in our thought process and psyche. So when we face resistance and road blocks in our everyday lives, it awakens us to be more open, flexible, and accommodative, and more accepting of the present moment. It teaches us to live in yoga.

Mental Loops

The mind is hardwired to dwell on defeating, negative thoughts over and over again; ruminating, regretting, wishing we could turn the clock back, rewrite the story, do things differently etc., all of which only leads to more *dukha* or suffering.

'We have between 60,000 and 80,000 thoughts a day—and many of them are the same thoughts we had yesterday, last week, and last year. The mind tends to get stuck in repetitive thought loops that squeeze out the possibility for new ideas and inspiration.'[4]

—Deepak Chopra

The nature of the mind is such that it is stuck like a broken recorder, playing and replaying the parts of our lives that cause us most anguish. We could have 90 per cent of our life working and 10 per cent that is not working, and yet our minds would be completely focused on the 10 per cent that doesn't work!

Brain scans of people recently out of a relationship have revealed that social pain (the emotional pain from a breakup or rejection) and physical pain share the same neural pathways. Scientists found that the same parts of the brain lit up when individuals looked at pictures of their partners or experienced physical pain but not when they looked at a friend's pictures. In further support of the overlap between physical and social pain, a study titled 'Acetaminophen Reduces Social Pain: Behavioural and Neural Evidence' concluded that Tylenol (an over-the-counter medication for physical pain) has been shown to reduce emotional pain! 'Acetaminophen reduces behavioural and neural responses associated with the pain of social rejection, demonstrating substantial overlap between social and physical pain.'[5]

4 Deepak Chopra, 5 Ways Meditation Can Make You Happier and More Successful at Work.' LinkedIn, July 19, 2013, https://www.linkedin.com/pulse/20130718224205-75054000-5-ways-meditation-can-make-you-happier/

5 C. Nathan DeWall et al., 'Acetaminophen Reduces Social Pain: Behavioral and Neural Evidence', *Psychological Science* 21, issue 7 (2010): 931–7.

The effect was also evident in brain scans. When feelings of rejection were induced, the part of the brain associated with physical pain lit up in participants who didn't take Tylenol. Those who took Tylenol showed significantly less activity in that part of the brain. 'Acetaminophen reduced neural responses to social rejection in brain regions previously associated with distress caused by social pain and the affective component of physical pain (dorsal anterior cingulate cortex, anterior insula)'.

There may be an evolutionary reason for this. The function of pain is to alert the person to physical danger or harm so they can take protective action. In the animal kingdom, one's chances of avoiding predators are much higher as part of a group than alone, therefore social rejection may have been an actual threat to physical survival for our early ancestors. If this is the case, it might partially explain how difficult it is for many people to let go of their ex-partners and move on. So getting through a breakup is as much a physical process as an emotional one.

The brain controls the body, and being under stress can trigger a cascade of effects: the release of stress hormones like cortisol and epinephrine affect the heart, the digestive system, and even the immune system.

- Too much cortisol in the brain sends blood to the major muscle groups. They tense up, ready to respond to the threat (fight or flight). As a result, our muscles swell, giving rise to headaches, a stiff neck and tightness in the chest.
- To ensure that the muscles have an adequate blood supply, cortisol diverts blood away from the digestive system. This can cause stomach troubles such as cramps, diarrhea or appetite loss.
- When stress hormones run rampant, the immune system can struggle, increasing vulnerability to bugs and illnesses.

- Breakups activate the area of the brain that processes craving and addiction.
- When your body's levels of dopamine, norepinephrine, and serotonin plummet during the later stages of a breakup, one very literally suffers from despair and resignation.
- Evidence also suggest that the almond-shaped amygdala in the brain is involved in feelings of separation distress, sadness, and, more generally, emotional memory.

The Antidote

Meditation is a powerful practice for going beyond habitual, conditioned thought patterns and reactions into a state of expanded awareness, which is the field of all potentiality and creativity. It lends clarity and elevates the mind to an insightful space.

Some Scientific Studies

Studies show that regular meditative practice can change structures in the brain. In 2011, a team led by Harvard-affiliated researchers at Massachusetts General Hospital (MGH) reported the results of their study, 'Mindfulness practice leads to increases in regional brain gray matter density'.[6]

For the study, magnetic resonance (MR) images were taken of the brain structure of 16 study participants two weeks before and after they took part in the eight-week Mindfulness-Based Stress Reduction (MBSR) Program at the University of Massachusetts Center for Mindfulness. In addition to weekly meetings that included the practice of mindfulness meditation, which focuses on non-judgmental awareness of sensations, feelings, and states of mind, participants received audio recordings for guided

6 Britta K. Hölzel et al., 'Mindfulness Practice Leads to Increase in Regional Brain Gray Matter Density', *Psychiatry Research* 191, issue 1 (2011): 36–43.

meditation practice and were asked to keep track of how much time they practiced each day. A set of MR brain images was also taken of a control group of non-meditators over a similar time interval. Meditation group participants reported spending an average of 27 minutes each day practicing mindfulness exercises, and their responses to a mindfulness questionnaire indicated significant improvements compared with pre-participation responses.

The analysis of MR images, which focused on areas where meditation-associated differences were seen in earlier studies, found increased grey matter density in the hippocampus, known to be important for learning and memory, and in structures associated with self-awareness, compassion, and introspection. Participant-reported reductions in stress were also correlated with decreased grey matter density in the amygdala, known as the anxiety, stress and fear structure of the brain.

A landmark study, 'Meditation experience is associated with increased cortical thickness'[7] discovered that meditators had much more density, thickness, and neural activity within their 'left pre-frontal cortex'—just like Albert Einstein. Increased thickness in this 'king of all brain regions could mean far less anxiety and depression, improved decision making, stronger willpower, more success, more processing power, better health, etc. for the meditators.' What's more, they also found that the more years of meditation experience a participant had under his/her belt, the greater the overall size of their super-beneficial prefrontal cortex.

A study, 'The Unique Brain Anatomy of Meditation Practitioners. Alterations In Cortical Gyrification',[8] by the

7 Sara W. Lazar et al., 'Meditation Experience is Associated With Increased Cortical Thickness', *NeuroReport* 16, issue 17 (2005): 1893–97.

8 Eileen Luders et al., 'The Unique Brain Anatomy of Meditation Practitioners: Alterations in Cortical Gyrification', *Frontiers in Human Neuroscience* 6, issue 34 (2012), https://www.ncbi.nlm.nih.gov/pmc/articles/PMC3289949/

University of California, Los Angeles (UCLA) found that the long-term meditators have larger amounts of gyrification ('folding' of the cortex, which may allow the brain to process information faster) than people who do not meditate. Further, a direct correlation was found between the amount of gyrification and the number of meditation years, possibly providing further proof of the brain's neuroplasticity or ability to adapt to environmental changes.

Another study, 'Bridging the hemispheres in meditation: thicker callosal regions and enhanced fractional anisotropy (FA) in long-term practitioners',[9] by the UCLA School of Medicine found that the meditators' 'corpus callosum'—the Grand Central Station-like cable of nerves connecting the brain hemispheres—was remarkably stronger, thicker, and more well-connected than those of non-meditators. This bridge-like structure is very helpful in getting your brain halves to communicate with each other. When both of your brain hemispheres are harmonized, you have increased focus, deeper thought, more creativity, optimized mental health, better memory, and clearer thinking, just to name a few benefits.

So the evidence is beginning to be gathered on the benefits of meditation, not merely on a superficial temporary level, but as having lasting structural changes in the brain itself.

While we are all comfortable with the known, it is the mysteries of the unknown that hold the secrets to both the universe and our own selves. This is the realm of expansion and the key to expanding into our greatest possibilities, our highest selves.

9 Eileen Luders et al. 'Bridging the Hemispheres in Meditation: Thicker Callosal Regions and Enhanced Fractional Anisotropy (FA) in Long-Term Practitioners', *NeuroImage* 61, issue, 1 (2012): 181–87.

Practice

1. **Rewire your brain**: Change patterns. Change patterns. Change patterns. Start something new: a new exercise routine, a reading pattern of a new book every week, a focus on diet and eating healthy which will lead to new interests and exploring new aisles in the grocery store.
2. **Open your mind**: Listen to motivating talks; it could be world leaders, spiritual teachers, or TED talks, just as long as you can resonate with it and it leaves you feeling inspired about your life and path.
3. **Question your own core beliefs**: Sometimes our own core beliefs, unconsciously adopted even as a child, limit us from living our best lives. 'First you make your beliefs and then your beliefs make you', says Marissa Peers, world renowned therapist and bestselling author. So question the beliefs you hold in your life as you unconciously live them out.
4. **Travel:** Take breaks and travel as often as you can. Being in different places with different people offers you an instant shift in perception.
5. **Identify with a higher calling**: Your life should be bigger than you. Whatever our job, it is always possible to give a little bit more, infuse a little more humanity, a little more love, and touch lives positively. It truly brings the greatest satisfaction.

Asanas: Hip-Opening

The 'foot behind the head' series of poses require great rotation and flexibility at the hip along with good strength of the paraspinal muscles. The effort taken towards accomplishing this pose embodies our commitment to take conscious effort to release our suffering and to move forward stronger, with greater clarity and wisdom.

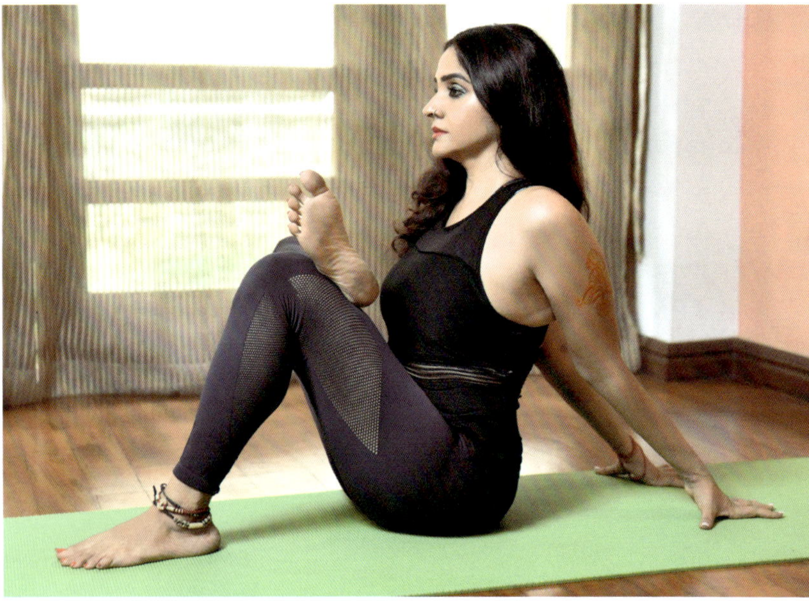

Seated *Kapotasana*

1. Sit on the mat with your legs stretched out in front of you.
2. Place your right foot on your left thigh just behind the left knee.
3. Bend your left knee, bringing your right foot towards your chest. Keep your hands behind you and press down through the palms to keep your chest lifted and heart open.

This helps to develop external rotation and opens the hips, a requirement for the foot behind the head series.

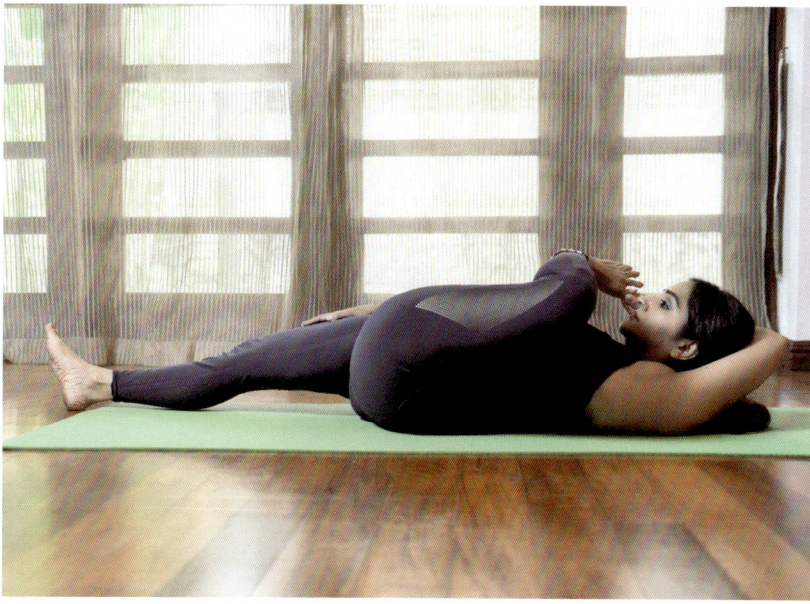

Suptapadangustasana

1. Lie on your back on the mat. Bend both your legs, keeping your feet on the floor. Externally rotate your right leg, bend your knee, and place your right foot just below the left knee. Make sure that the toes of your right foot are pointing upward (dorsi-flexed foot) rather than pointing to the left side (plantar-flexed foot).
2. Bring your left knee towards your chest, which strongly works on opening the right outer hips. You can either stay here by hugging your left thigh, or, if this feels comfortable, you can move into the next option.
3. Bring your right hand over your head and catch hold of your right foot beside the left side of your face. Slowly straighten your left leg down onto the mat.

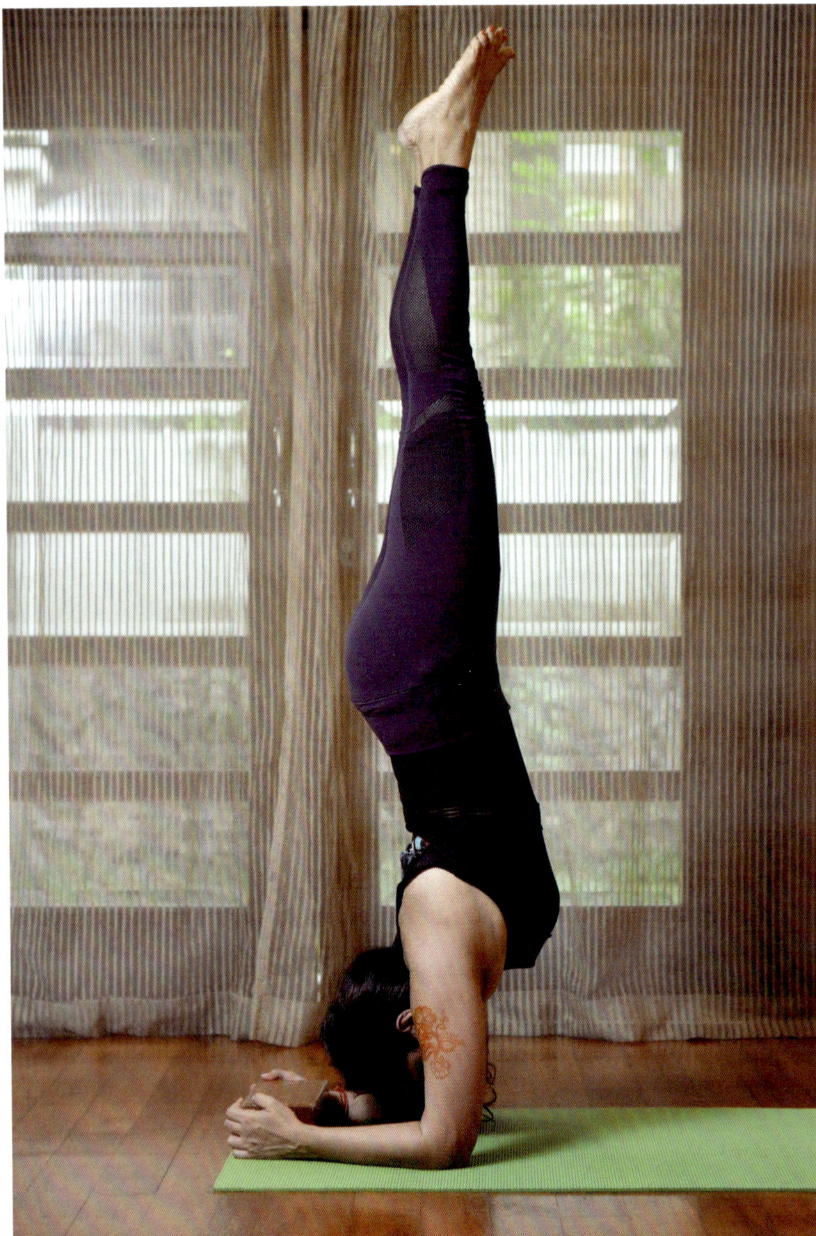

Artistic Pose: *Pincha Mayurasana* or Forearm Handstand

The Grandeur of *Vairagya*

> *The senses are mere instruments of the mind; they cannot act by themselves. It is the mind and discrimination that must be freed from enslavement.*[1]
>
> —Sri Sri Paramahansa Yogananda

Abhayasa and *Vairagya*

Sage Vyasa compares consciousness to a *chitta nadi* (river) which can flow in two directions—towards *kalyana* (auspiciousness, beauty) or towards *papa* (inauspiciousness). When the river is inclined towards *viveka* (discriminatory wisdom), the flow is towards *kalyana,* eventually leading to what Vyasa terms *kaivalya praghbara* (reservoir of liberation). When inclined towards *a-viveka* (lack of discriminatory wisdom) it leads us towards *papa* (inauspiciousness) and ends in *samsara pragbhara* (reservoir of worldly entanglements).

An important quality to stem the flow towards samsara is the *abhyasa* (practice) of *vairagya,* or detachment. In fact, even in the

1 Paramahansa Yogananda, *God Talks With Arjuna: The Bhagavad Gita* (Kolkata: Yagoda Satsanga Society of India, 2011).

Bhagavad Gita, Lord Krishna imparts the exact same techniques to controlling consciousness—*abhyasa* and *vairagya.*

The very meaning of *vairagya* (which comes from *vi* and *ranj*) is 'devoid of colouring'. *Vairagya* is therefore the process of de-coloring the shield of consciousness from judgment, prejudices, labels, conditions, demands and desires to translucence and eventually, transparency.

One of the primary causes of suffering is deep attachment. But rest assured that *vairagya* is not about detaching from the good things in life as people assume. It is about withdrawing from the currents of life that take us downward and sap our energy and joy, so that we can experience freedom from bondage. So before exploring *vairagya* or detachment, we have to look at it in the context of its counterpart, *raga* or deep attachment.

But really, is it possible to live without being attached? The human mind has the amazing ability to be attached to just about everything! The side of the bed we sleep on, our houses, cars, our patterns of going to the gym, patterns of food and drink (start the day with coffee!), yoga class, not to mention Facebook, WhatsApp, video games, money and of course the many relationships we have in our lives with people, children, dogs, and cats etc. Need I go on?

So let us first be aware of our attachments. What are our deepest attachments? What situations or persons are we bound to? We don't have to look very far; in fact, we just have to look at the different areas in our lives—people and situations that affect us or cause us pain, and there we will find them. Are you in a bad mood if you don't get your morning coffee? Or when you notice that somebody has taken your favourite space in yoga class? Or if your usual parking lot in the gym is occupied? Are you affected if a particular person doesn't smile at you when you enter the room? There lies your attachment.

Are All Attachments Bad?

It comes down to the degree of attachment. If the attachment is something that doesn't affect you when you are deprived of it, then the attachment is not an unhealthy one. Such as, if your parking lot is taken, you just park in the next available lot. But if it takes you to a point of rage, where you are plotting to puncture the hapless guy's car tyres, then you know there's something not quite right there. Similarly, if we have a liking for sweets, can we give them up even if we are diagnosed with diabetes? Are we down in the dumps and contemplating ending our lives if a person doesn't call us? When attachment turns shades of obsessive compulsive, it is certainly unhealthy and needs to be looked into.

How easily can we give it up? How do we react to the 'not having of it'? Therein lies the answer. When it colours our mind with shaking rage, violence, overwhelming sadness and depression, anxiety, or thoughts of revenge and death; then we know, we have to take many steps back, make drastic changes in our lives, and release ourselves from the situation. This allows us to reclaim our power and find our inner alignment. And only we can do that. Like the famous phrase mentioned in the Bhagavad Gita, chapter 6, verse 6, *'uddharet atmanatmanam'*— 'We have to lift ourselves by ourselves'.[2]

Drshtanu shravika vishaya vitrshnasya vashikara sanjna vairagyam

When objects by way of being seen and heard lose their hold on the consciousness by way of the yogi's mastery over them, that state is vairagya.[3]

—Patanjali's *Yoga Sutras*, chapter 1, sutra 15

2 Paramahansa Yogananda, *God talks to Arjuna: The Bhagavad Gita* (Kolkata: Yagoda Satsanga Society of India, 2011).

3 Manoj Kaimal, *Making Patanjali Palatable* (Manoj Kaimal, 2008).

The word that fascinated me was *vashikara,* or mastery.

With deep attachment comes a thirst, longing, craving, an almost obsessive need to have a certain end point, a specific outcome or a desired condition met. *Vairagya* is the *vashikara* or the mastery of this deep thirst. So how does one go about releasing oneself from the clutches of this attachment to a child, partner, lover, job, house, money, or pet? How does one find a release from the suffering that inevitably follows this? There are four stages in the process:

First, we need to develop an awareness of ***yatha mana***. Where is the mind? Most of us live in such a deep state of unconsciousness that we just flow with the mind wherever it likes to go. Only when we are in a state of deep pain and suffering do we begin to assess how we got there in the first place! Hence, it is good to be aware of the mind during different parts of the day, and of the different states of the mind as well—its restless nature, its constant flitting from person to person or object to object, its reactions to different people and situations, its tendency to get obsessive-compulsive about one person or a situation.

Vyatireka: With awareness, we develop a clarity about our thought processes, our mental tendencies and our patterns—that the same person or situation is always there at the back of our mind, that we always reach for the same food or drink at a particular time, that we always react in the same manner to a particular person's action, that the triggers that set us off are the same. Thus, we have clarity over the destabilizing factors within our mind. The more clarity dawns, the more we get unstuck.

Ekendriya: We then come to realize that we have to stop pointing fingers at other people, events or situations and take back our power by assuming responsibility for our lives. Our minds create situations and, by changing our perspective, we have the ability to release the situation too. Through continuous 'seeing', over a period of time, *viveka* or discriminative wisdom develops in us, enough to recognize when a particular thought, action or pattern stabilizes or destabilizes our minds. If we observe that it takes us downhill, and has been doing so over a period of time, we also become conscious of the power to make different choices in order to release that 'taking-us-downhill' pattern from our lives. We could go for a walk, change jobs, move cities, hit the gym, learn a new language, travel, or sign up for a class. We always have a choice.

Vashikara: As we continue gaining clarity, even previously desired objects will lose their hold over us. We then rest in mastery, in a perspective that we have chosen that is in alignment with our minds and lives.

Asana is Life: Transformation On and Off the Mat

Our asana practice provides us with a powerful opportunity in terms of time and space to objectively watch the mind and its gyrations—its sadness when we can't touch our toes in *uttanasana* (standing forward fold), our plummeting self-esteem if we can't lift up into *urdhva dhanurasana* (upward bow pose) and our neighbour can, our frustration at being unable to bend our leg behind our head. This objective witnessing of the mind lends us clear insights into the way our minds operate and where our thinking needs to be tweaked and adjusted. So, on the mat itself we could tell our minds, 'It's all right if I can't touch my toes just yet, the practice of asana is not about end points. It is about enjoying the journey'. Or as we watch our thoughts of envy as our neighbor does asanas that we struggle with, we could tell ourselves, 'I am inspired watching her do it. Our paths are not the same. I just began two months ago and she has been a regular for more than a year. With consistent practice my body too will be able to respond well. For now, let me just be grateful and appreciate what my body is able to do'.

Thus, the work begins on the mat where we develop consciousness of our thoughts and our ability to tweak them to a more optimistic state in our asana practice. Our minds on the mat and off the mat are not separate. Asana is life, and the same attitude that we express in asana practice is generally what we hold in the rest of our lives too. Slowly, this capacity of 'awareness of our thoughts and states of mind' that we consciously develop in our asana practice over time permeates into our thinking and colours the rest of our lives too. So when we face challenges in our lives or come across road blocks per se—we don't clinch the deal we worked so hard for, we don't get that raise or promotion we believed was due to us, we have a miscarriage, a relationship ends etc.—instead of being drowned in depression, anxiety or rage, we have the ability to consciously shift perspective and sooth ourselves into a more optimistic, hopeful state of mind which then gives birth to a different tone of thought that shifts our state of mind.

But if we have never consciously practiced it before, it is near impossible to suddenly make this mental shift in our everyday life. Our minds simply drown in the avalanche of turbulent emotions. So the immense value of cultivating and strengthening this ability to shift our perspective to a broader, softer and more accommodative approach in our asana practice, where the stakes are not so high and emotions not so raw, cannot be over-emphasized. Asana practice thus becomes the tool by which we stretch our minds from tightness, sadness and disappointment to faith, hope and optimism, and eventually to higher states of gratitude and appreciation.

Keep Expanding, Keep Growing

When we are deeply attached, our world closes and our focus narrows. Our whole lives are consciously or unconsciously built around the one person, job, or eating and lifestyle pattern. We stop trying different things, exploring, or doing things spontaneously out of instinct. In short, we stop growing and get stuck. So the process of getting unstuck requires us to open our worlds, broaden our lives. The key is to deeply seek freedom in every fibre of our being. We should want to release ourselves from the tyranny of bondage to a debilitating pattern—from an eating pattern that keeps us unhealthy and overweight, a relationship pattern that eats away at our sanity, a job situation that attacks our self-respect, to a drinking pattern that destroys our life and the lives of the people around us.

Take Responsibility

The ultimate responsibility for the state of our minds and our lives is ours and ours alone. It lies with us. We cannot change conditions outside of us nor can we control the actions of other persons and situations. Things happen. The only control we have is the ability to shift our perspective and our response to events that unfold in our lives.

As we continue with the inner work, we have to realize that while there are outer situations that disturb us, ultimately it is our own mind, out of its own conditioning and mental projections, that expects, reacts, judges and condemns. We could be perfectly justified in blaming someone or something else—a person, the country, the economy, our parents, or our teachers, but it takes us nowhere. We remain in the same place, with the same stories. The more responsibility we assume for the state of our minds and our lives, the more empowered we become to effect change in our lives.

Inner Work

The most important capacity we have is the ability to shift our perspective and change our story. We have the capacity to choose our focus. The power lies within us. We can choose to see the learning in the experience, to know that each experience only throws more clarity on the working of our own minds and its weaknesses, strengths and desires. From this, we come to the realization that if we can see the bigger picture of our lives, we will realize that the dots connect; that each disappointment that we experienced only gave birth to greater clarity and wisdom, and took us towards the unfolding of the highest expression of our selves.

Taking responsibility is a big word. We have to see that it is our own mind that closes us off, believes that we have no other option—that we cannot survive without this job, this drink, this smoke, this food, this relationship or marriage. It is fear that keeps us small, bound and limited. Yet once we acknowledge it, we find the courage to push past it, go beyond the borders of our comfort zones, and taste true freedom.

'I learned that courage was not the absence of fear, but the triumph over it. The brave man is not he who does not feel afraid, but he who conquers that fear.'[4]

—Nelson Mandela

What I found very effective in my own life, was the concept of 'aligning to a higher value'. Once our mind is aligned to a higher value—like love and respect for ourselves, of wanting to be our best possible self at all levels of existence, or living selflessly, it

4 Nelson Mandela, *Long Walk to Freedom* (Johannesburg, South Africa: Macdonald Purnell, 1994).

provides the strength to release ourselves from the grip of other needs and compulsions, however strong they may be. Hard though the path may be, we have the satisfaction of gaining ourselves—our self-love and respect, connecting to our own power, and living an aligned and authentic life.

We have to keep faith in the magic of the universe.

'Faith is the bird that feels the light and sings when the dawn is still dark.'[5]

—Rabindranath Tagore

Through continuous inner work, and by sifting through our thoughts, day by day, we strengthen our ability to consciously shift our focus to areas of our lives that work, that bring us joy and fulfillment. And no effort in that direction is ever wasted. Every conscious attempt is a process that strengthens the fresh neural pathways that we are creating in the brain which, in time, make these pathways stronger.

We all have to become alchemists; transmuting our wounds, our losses, our disappointments, our sorrows into a treasure trove of understanding and wisdom!

Practice

1. Be in conscious touch with your emotions. Observe areas in your life that repeatedly cause you pain. Write them down.
2. Explore the cause. Though we would like to blame someone or something outside of us, it will usually be some deep attachment or expectation that we have.
3. Take responsibility for your pain. Explore and weigh your

5 From Rabindranath Tagore's poem, 'Fireflies'.

options. Know that you always have a choice in how you want to feel and live.

4. Take a step back and create some space from the situation so you can be more objective before you take a decision. It also allows you to look at life from a larger perspective.
5. As you begin to consciously tune in to your inner guidance, you will know the right path for you.

Asanas: Inversions

Inversions literally shift our perspective of a situation upside down! This is so that we can come a little unstuck and broaden our perspective. We have to learn to look at a situation not just through our eyes, but also from someone else's point of view and become more accommodative in the process.

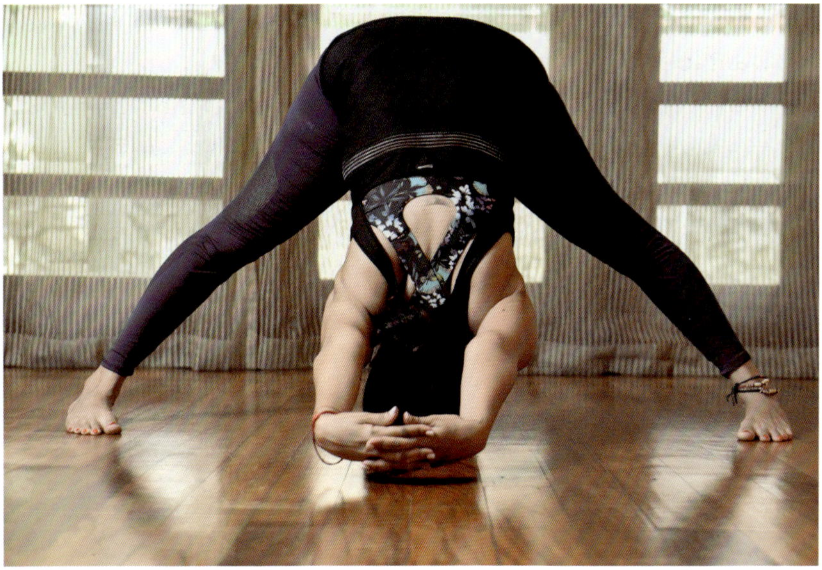

Prasaritapadottanasana 3: Standing Wide-Leg Forward Fold

1. Stand with your feet wide apart and the inner edges of your feet parallel to each other. Clasp your hands behind you, fingers interlaced.
2. Inhale, roll your shoulders back, and lift your chest. Exhale as you fold your torso.
3. Keep working on moving your upper arms away from your upper back and towards the floor.
4. Hold for 5–10 breaths.
5. Inhale, press down through the feet as you rise up. Exhale and release your arms.

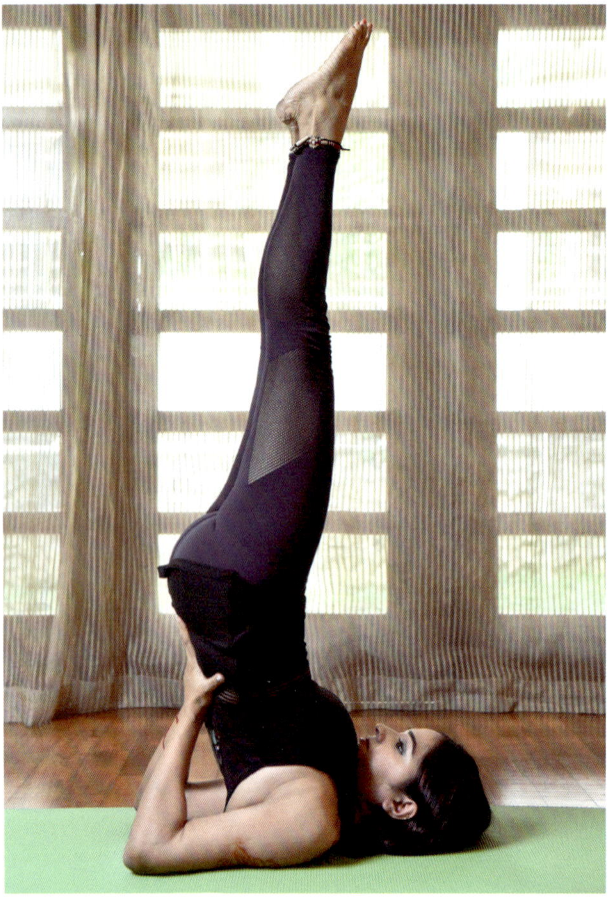

Sarvangasana, Halasana, Padmasarvangasana: Shoulder Stand, Plough Pose, Variations of Lotus in Shoulder Stand

1. Lie down on your back.
2. Lift your hips and legs up off the floor and support your back with your palms, keeping your elbows on the floor. Wriggle your shoulders and elbows in, and try to walk your hands as far up your back and towards your shoulder blades as possible. Keep lifting your back ribs upward, away from the floor, and stretch your legs and feet upward. Make sure the edges of your big toes are touching each other. This is *sarvangasana*. Stay for 5–10 breaths.

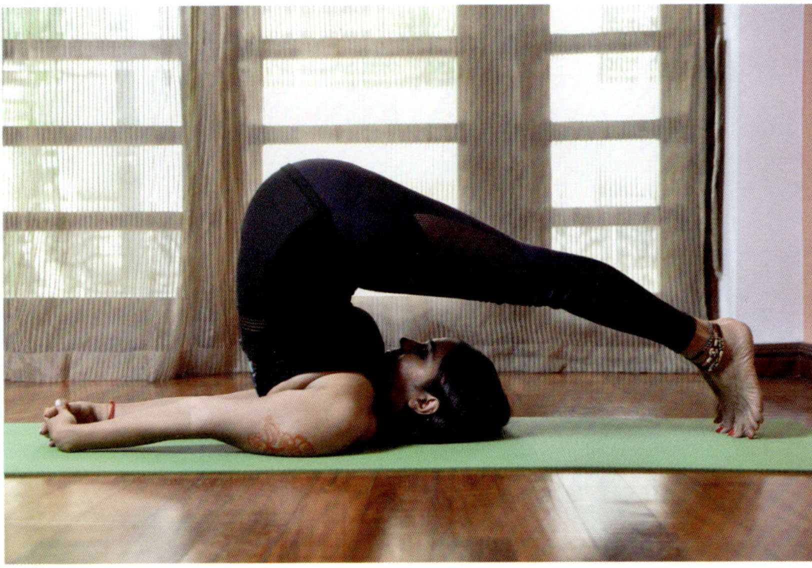

3. Slowly bend your legs and knees towards your face. If your neck and back feel comfortable, slowly straighten your legs and feet towards the floor. This is *halasana*. Stay for 5–10 breaths.

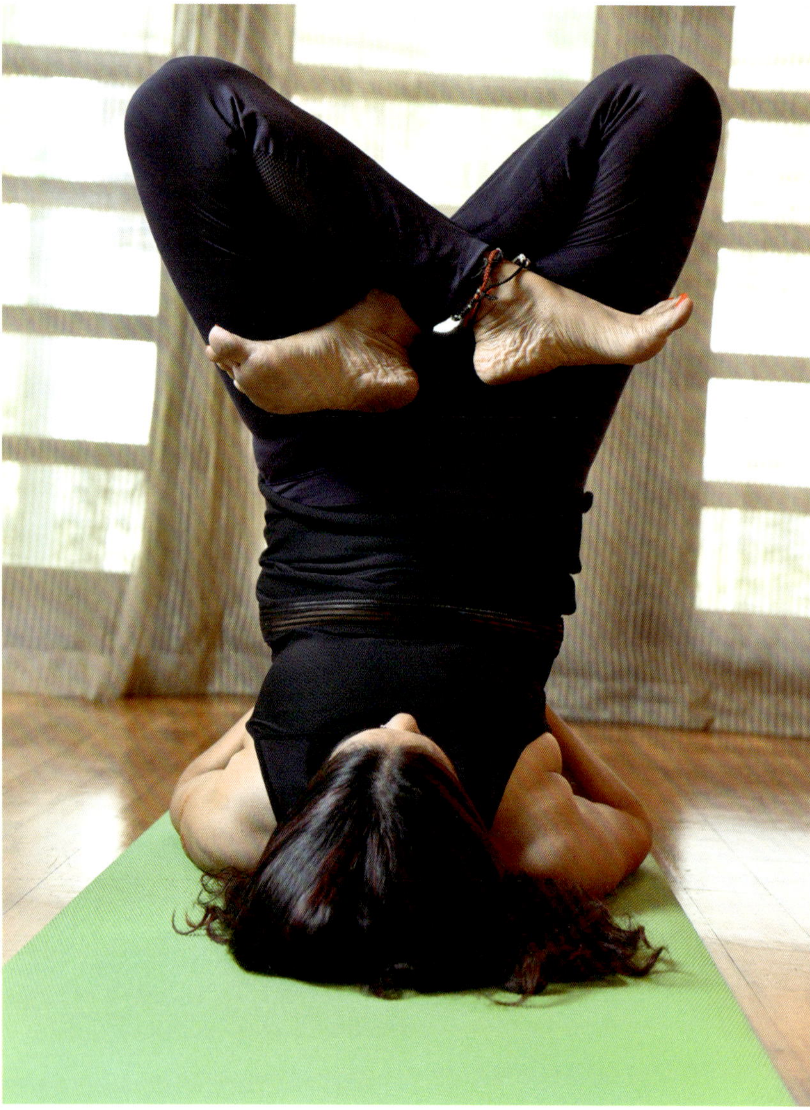

4. If your hips are open, and you can do regular *padmasana* on the floor, then in *sarvangasana*, you can bend one knee and bring your heel towards the opposite hip crease. You can use your hand to adjust your foot. Bend your other knee to lower your heel towards the opposite hip crease. This is *padma sarvangasana*.

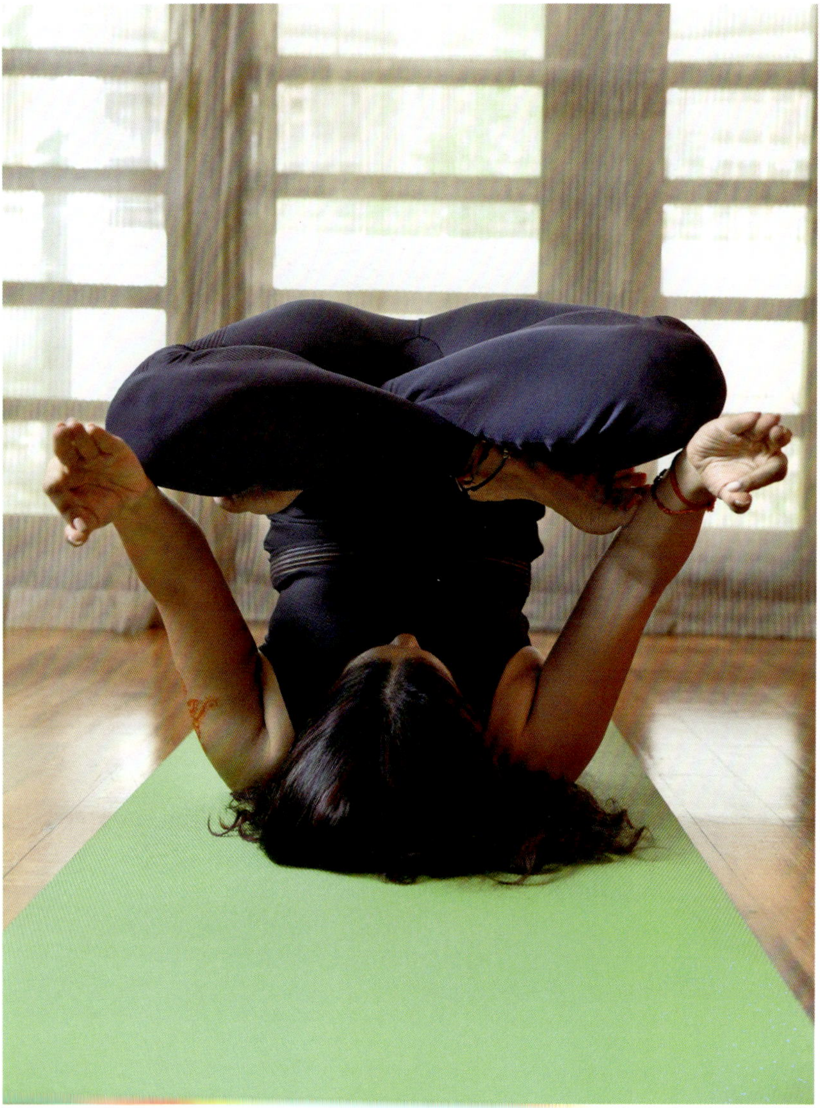

If you would like to explore further, lift your arms up and place your hands against your knees, keeping your thighs parallel to the floor. Find your balance.

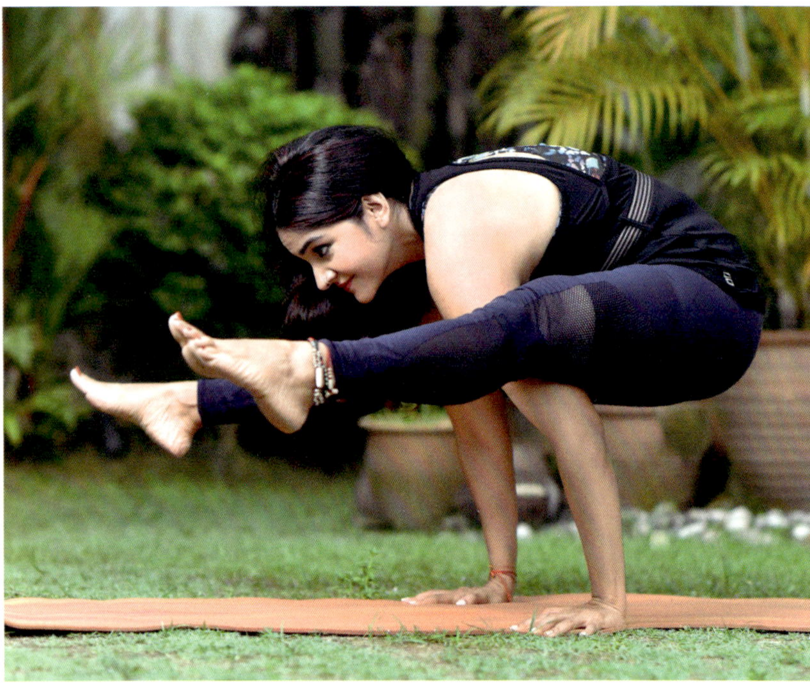

Artistic Pose: *Tittibhasana* or Firefly Pose

Alignment

It is through the alignment of the body that I discovered the alignment of my mind, self, and intelligence.[1]

—Guruji B.K.S. Iyengar

While a lot of focus is placed on the alignment of the body, the ultimate alignment that we seek is the alignment of the mind with universal intelligence. For this, awareness is the key, and we work by sifting through our minds—thought by thought, emotion by emotion, state of mind by state of mind.

As I begin my class, I first ask my students to direct their attention to their minds; to be aware of, to observe and be present to what goes on in their minds.

Where is your mind? What occupies your mind? Is it a person or a situation? Acknowledge that.

1 B.K.S. Iyengar, *Light on Life: The Yoga Journey to Wholesomeness, Inner Peace, and Ultimate Freedom.* (USA: Rodale Inc., 2005).

From there, I direct them to shift their focus to the different parts of the body.

Sit with your spine long, chest open, shoulders rolled back, face relaxed, eyes closed. Be aware of the sense of touch; keep the outer edges of your feet against the mat. Explore that sense of touch. Is the mat rough? Smooth? There is no judgment. Nothing is right or wrong. Only an awareness of, 'what is'. Become aware of the inner edges of your feet. What can you feel? Is it your inner thigh? Is it your calves? Simply observe.

Become aware of the sit bones. Feel the pressure of the sit bones against the mat. As you direct your awareness to the sit bone area, there will be some insights, some learning. Are you sitting at the front of the sit bones, the back, or the middle? Explore. Can you shift to the middle of the sit bones? Become aware of your spine, keep your spine long. Become aware of the chest. Deliberately draw your shoulder blades towards each other so your chest is open. Sense the expansiveness in your chest.

Become aware of your arms. Explore which part of your arm is against your knees or your thighs. Is it your forearms or is it your wrist? Is it your palm or the back of your palm? Become aware of your neck. Is it in line with your spine? Become aware of your face. Relax your jaw, the area around your eyes, the skin of the forehead and temples. Let your whole face completely relax.

Once they do that, they are guided to shift their focus to their breath.

Shift your focus to your breath. Feel the breath flow in and out as you inhale and exhale. Feel the sense of touch as your breath flows. The breath always operates in the present. Now the breath becomes our atha, *our present experience.*

The more we connect to and deepen our capacity to consciously shift our attention, from whatever occupies our minds, to remain stable on our breath, the more we strengthen the capacity of our mind to make conscious shifts; from thoughts that bring sadness and grief to thoughts that are more neutral. And this is the vital capacity that ultimately helps us to consciously create our lives and maintain the state of our minds in positive, inspired grooves of thinking.

In asana practice, they are similarly guided to shift their focus to their bodies.

Feel the resistance of the hamstrings in hanumanasana *(front split position), the tightening of the abdominal muscles, the contraction of the quadriceps and hip flexors in* navasana *(boat pose), the deep flexion of the spine and shoulders in* urdhva dhanurasana *(upward bow pose).*

While this process helps them to be present to their bodies, it ever-so methodically hones another huge capacity; the ultimate capacity to consciously direct our minds and shift our focus. This places the power squarely back in our hands, as we become magnificent creators of our reality as opposed to being victims and powerlessly reacting to people and situations.

Ultimately, life is perspective. As humans, we hold the trump card as we have the ability to choose our perspective.

But that powerful capacity comes from the degree to which we are aware of our thoughts, our emotions and the state of our minds. Most of the time, our minds are consumed in the story-self—in what happened to us, in what may happen, in the likely and unlikely scenarios that could unfold, in imagination, and in fantasy. So we get lost in a maze of thoughts and reactions. Why is life so unfair? Why are some people luckier than others? Why me? How could they do this to me and get away with it? How can I get back at them? Why did he smile at me? Why didn't he smile at me? You get my drift.

While driving, while studying, while going to sleep, on waking up, the questions and reactions and overreactions haunt our every waking moment. Emotions accompany those thoughts too; the sadness, the disbelief, and the disillusionment which slowly gives way to anger and rage. The scenarios, the dialogues, the counter dialogues just keep repeating like a broken record in our heads until we realize that we don't want to live like this! We understand that it affects our physical and mental health, and its toxicity seeps into our every relationship and every aspect of life, slowly eating away everything that is beautiful within us.

We have to know that ultimately, it is not stress that kills us, but our own unique perspective of stress.

But simply knowing is not enough. We have to ACT. Instead of being at the mercy of the capricious monkey mind and allowing the state of our minds to be dictated, we have to call upon our deep capacity to direct our attention and shift our focus to where we choose, towards parts of our lives that work! And that is the most powerful inner capacity we can develop.

This calls for immense strength of mind to overcome its inherent whimsical nature that operates on likes and dislikes. It calls for a deep objective awareness of the direction of our thoughts, actions, emotions and the resulting state of mind. It calls for the continuous honing of our ability to shift our attention to neutral thoughts or areas of our lives that work. With repeated practice, this capacity strengthens and generates a momentum to keep the mind in positive neural pathways.

So how can something as random as sitting and focusing on your breath or holding a yoga posture change the state of our emotions and mind? The answer lies again in neuroplasticity, for as we engage in a particular behaviour over and over again, this can lead to changes in our brain structure. The brain is plastic and the neurons can change the way they talk and communicate to each other over time.

> *In our everyday lives, if we intentionally set out to learn new things or do familiar things in new ways (such as commuting to work via a new route or taking the bus instead of a car), we effectively rewire our brains and improve them. A physical workout builds muscle; a mental workout creates new synapses to strengthen the neural network.*
>
> *The bottom line is that we are not 'hardwired'. Our brains are incredibly resilient; the marvelous process of neuroplasticity gives you the capability, in your thoughts, feelings, and actions, to develop in any direction you choose.*[2]
>
> —Deepak Chopra and Rudolph E. Tanzi

Through MRI scans of the brain, studies have been conducted that detect an increase in grey matter on corresponding parts of the brain that are activated through specific skills or tasks. A famous study, 'Acquiring "the Knowledge" of London's Layout Drives

2 Deepak Chopra and Rudolph E. Tanzi, *Super Brain: Unleashing the Explosive Power of Your Mind to Maximize Health, Happiness, and Spiritual Well-Being* (London: Rider Books, 2012).

Structural Brain Changes',[3] was conducted on London taxi drivers. It supports the increasing evidence that even in adult life, learning can change the structure of the brain, offering encouragement for lifelong learning and the potential for rehabilitation after brain damage. The research suggested that structural brain differences may have been acquired through the experience of navigating, and to accommodate the internal representation of London. At the end of three–four years, they found a greater volume of grey matter in the posterior hippocampus, which is responsible for spatial memory in those trainees that qualified as taxi drivers, than they had before they started their training.

We connect to this capacity from the very start of our yoga class, when we consciously shift our attention from the many thoughts and ongoing debates in our minds to the *atha* practice, where we become present to our body.

That is the yoga practice. And it doesn't happen overnight. For years we have been slaves to the mind, catering to its every whim—what it likes to eat, what it doesn't like to eat, regardless of whether it is good for us or not; whether it likes to go to the gym or to stay home and vegetate, regardless of what is good for the body; whether it likes to read inspirational books or watch junk TV serials and flip from Facebook to WhatsApp, regardless of what is good!

Every time we take a seat on our mats and observe our thoughts and the state of our minds, every time we direct the mind to stay on the body in asana practice or to shift the focus to the breath and count, say, a 1000 or 5000 breaths, the underlying thrust is to strengthen our capacity to direct our minds and shift

---

3 Katherine Woollett and Eleanor A. Maguire, 'Acquiring "the Knowledge" of London's Layout Drives Structural Brain Changes', *Current Biology* 21, no. 24 (2011): 2109–14.

our attention to stay where WE choose. That capacity is the KEY to release from suffering, and it is the path to freedom.

Develop a Genuine Interest

The key to converting this practice from a tussle with the mind and trying to wrestle it to the ground is to develop a genuine interest in cultivating a deeper, intimate connection with the body and the breath. The mind has the ability to stay on whatever it is interested in. When we go to watch a movie, if the story line or the character grips our imagination, then we have no problem in keeping our attention focused on the screen in front of us for three hours!

Neurologically too, it is the release of the neurotransmitter dopamine that locks in our attention. Interestingly, what ensures the release of dopamine is interest! Dopamine is like the 'save button' in the brain. When dopamine is present during an event or experience, we remember it; when it is absent, nothing seems to stick. Some regions of the brain, referred to collectively as the *reward center,* are activated by dopamine and increase our motivation and interest in activities.

The more motivated and interested we are in an activity, the more dopamine is released and the better we remember it. The reward center helps us stay focused and repeat activities that were reinforced through positive outcomes—whether it is going back to our childhood where good things happened for us, reliving those magical moments in our lives, or even just remembering interesting information. Learning new and exciting information is the key to sustaining high levels of dopamine in the brain.

Releasing Trauma

We have to know that the mind, body and breath are all connected. Our every thought produces a resulting chemical reaction that floods our bloodstream and reflects in every cell of our body. When we are angry, agitated, or sense a threat, the body releases the hormones cortisol, adrenaline, and norepinephrine. When we are excited and happy, the body releases endorphins, dopamine, serotonin, and oxytocin.

> *This being so, emotions of the mind gets mirrored as muscular patterns in the tissues of the body. Repeated thoughts become habitual thought patterns, and habitual thought patterns become a physical postural pattern. So when we are stressed, it is reflected not merely in our mind and blood, but also as tension patterns along our muscles.*
>
> *And it is right here, through asana, from the tissues of the muscles, that we start the restoration of our nervous system into homeostasis. As we release the physiology of stress, the psychology of stress releases too.*
>
> —Manoj Kaimal

The Role of Asana - Aren't They Just Shapes?

Asana is the portal through which we connect to our *svarupa*, our true self, the deepest essence of ourselves; beyond the restlessness, beyond the agitations, beyond the frustrations, beyond the irritations, beyond our disappointments, beyond our perceived limitations, beyond the various identities of race, job, nationality, and relationships that we bind ourselves in, to reach our true limitless, boundless essence.

The Ultimate Alignment With Our Inner Selves

It is well known that asanas focus on the alignment of the body. But it is a lesser-known fact that the ultimate alignment is that of our minds and our lives with our true nature—what moves us, what inspires us, what we believe in, what brings meaning to our lives and how we live from that space. But it begins with the body.

As we are all infinite expressions of one universal energy, the more we are aligned to our true nature, the more this energy flows freely through us and expresses itself through our creativity and interactions.

My Journey

I am the first to admit that as far back as I can remember, I have been a seeker. I had no idea what it was that I was looking for; all I knew was that there was this void inside me that I was constantly trying to fill. This sense of incompleteness left me restless, discontented, anxious, and searching. I looked for validation from people and relationships. But the more I sought it from outside of myself, the more it eluded me. I began to read voraciously, I listened to spiritual talks, attended Vedanta and Bhagavad Gita classes. At some point yoga entered my life. In the beginning I did it because I felt good at the end of the class. But as time passed and trials tested me, I poured myself into my practice and derived my solace and strength from there. As my connection to myself deepened, the restlessness, the seeking, and the need to seek external validation became less and less. And as I continue to strengthen my inner connection and express myself authentically through my creative endeavours, the questions become fewer and the sense of void dissipates.

So while we seek and open our minds through whatever means available, we must earnestly seek that connection to ourselves, our centre, our core. And it is a conscious seeking. We can seek it through sitting with ourselves in silence every day, our connection with nature, our asana and other sitting practices, journaling, or whatever works for us. We must make it our priority to create the time and space in our lives to nurture and strengthen our inner connection, to own our power. For the ultimate relationship is with ourselves!

Practice

1. As you begin your yoga practice, consciously connect to your capacity to shift your focus—from your thoughts, to your body, and to your breath. The more you identify and work with this capacity, the more you strengthen it.
2. Identify patterns of thinking that makes you anxious or distressed. Whenever you find yourself thinking such thoughts, consciously shift the focus to something neutral—your breath, the sky, the touch of your sit bones on the chair.
3. During the day, make it a habit to consciously direct your attention to neutral activities—the touch of your feet on the ground as you walk, the rhythm of your arms as they swing, the touch of the breeze as it caresses your face, the energy of the kids as they run around in the playground.
4. Keep a gratitude journal where every morning you write 5–10 things that you are grateful for, and that have happened over the last 24 hours. It could be something as simple as having gratitude for a hot cup of coffee, a smile from a stranger or a pat of recognition from your boss. This way, you are consciously creating fresh neural pathways of appreciation and gratitude in the brain. Soon you will find that during the day, even unconsciously, the brain will be looking for things to enter in the journal, and you will be living life through the lens of gratitude.

Asanas: Strength

A lot of us go through life stuck in places, situations, relationships, jobs that we don't have the strength to release ourselves from, because we believe that we have no other choice. It takes great courage to first acknowledge where we are objectively, to see the fear, and to realize the untruths we tell ourselves and others, in order to be able to make different choices. Otherwise we continue to live shackled lives, never expressing our highest potential. Nor do we gain the freedom and strength that we seek in life, embodied through strong and challenging arm balances.

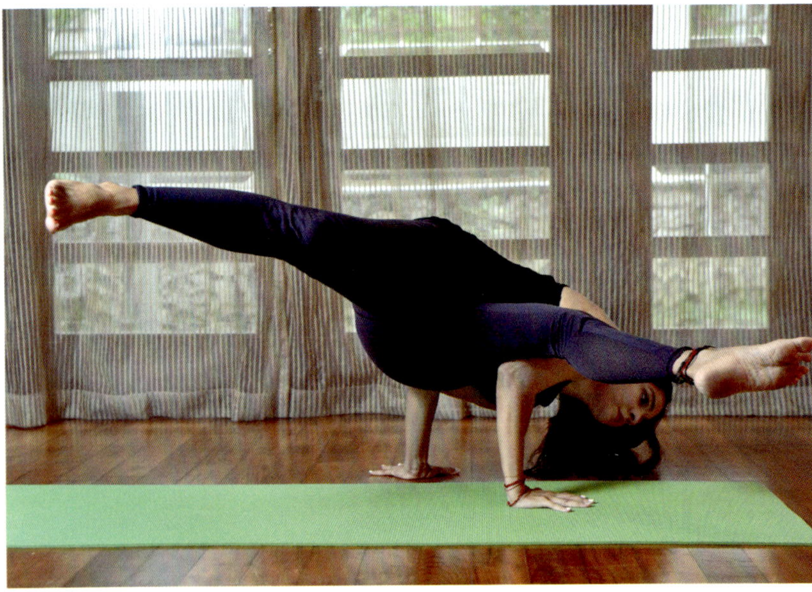

Parivrtta Eka Pada Koundinyasana

1. Come on to your hands and knees.
2. Take a step forward with your right foot.
3. Take your left upper arm across your right thigh and place both your palms on the floor, shoulder-widh apart.
4. Bend your arms as you lean your upper body to the right so that your navel comes in line with your palms.
5. Take your right foot off the floor and extend your right knee.
6. Lean further foward and raise your left leg off the floor as well.
7. Stay for a few breaths and change sides.

This is a challenging intermediate pose, and is best to be gradually built- up under the guidance of a teacher.

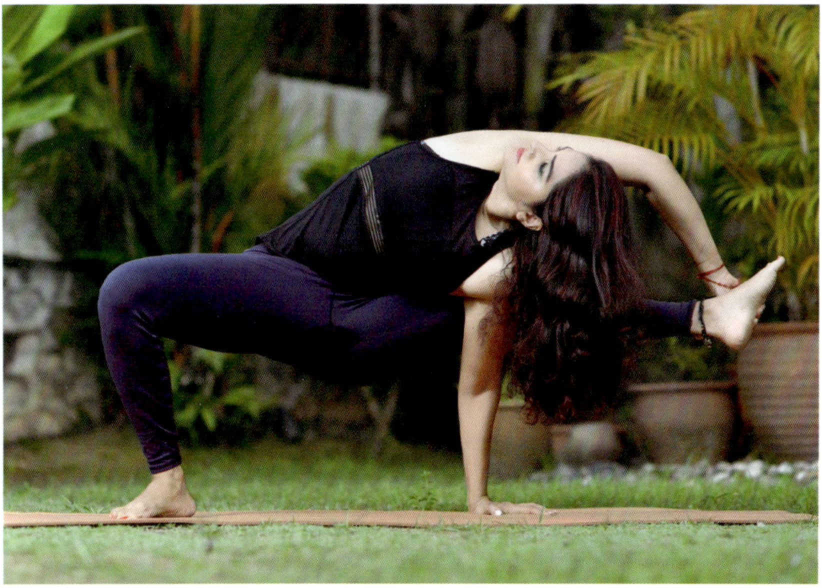

Mala Vishwamitrasana

1. Stand with your feet more than hip-width apart.
2. Slowly bend forward and place your hands on the floor. Bend your legs so that the buttocks come to the line of the knees.
3. From this position, take your right shoulder and upper arm behind your right calf and place your right hand just behind and beside your right foot.
4. Lean backward into your right hand, and, as you feel a lightness to your right foot, lift it off the floor.
5. Reach out with your left hand and catch hold of your right foot. Work on straightening your right leg against the resistance of your right upper arm, using the help of your left hand.
6. Rotate the ribs strongly upward and away from the floor.

Repeat on the other side.

As with *Parivrtta Eka Pada Koundinyasana*, this is also an intermediate pose, and you will be best served learning this under a teacher's supervision.

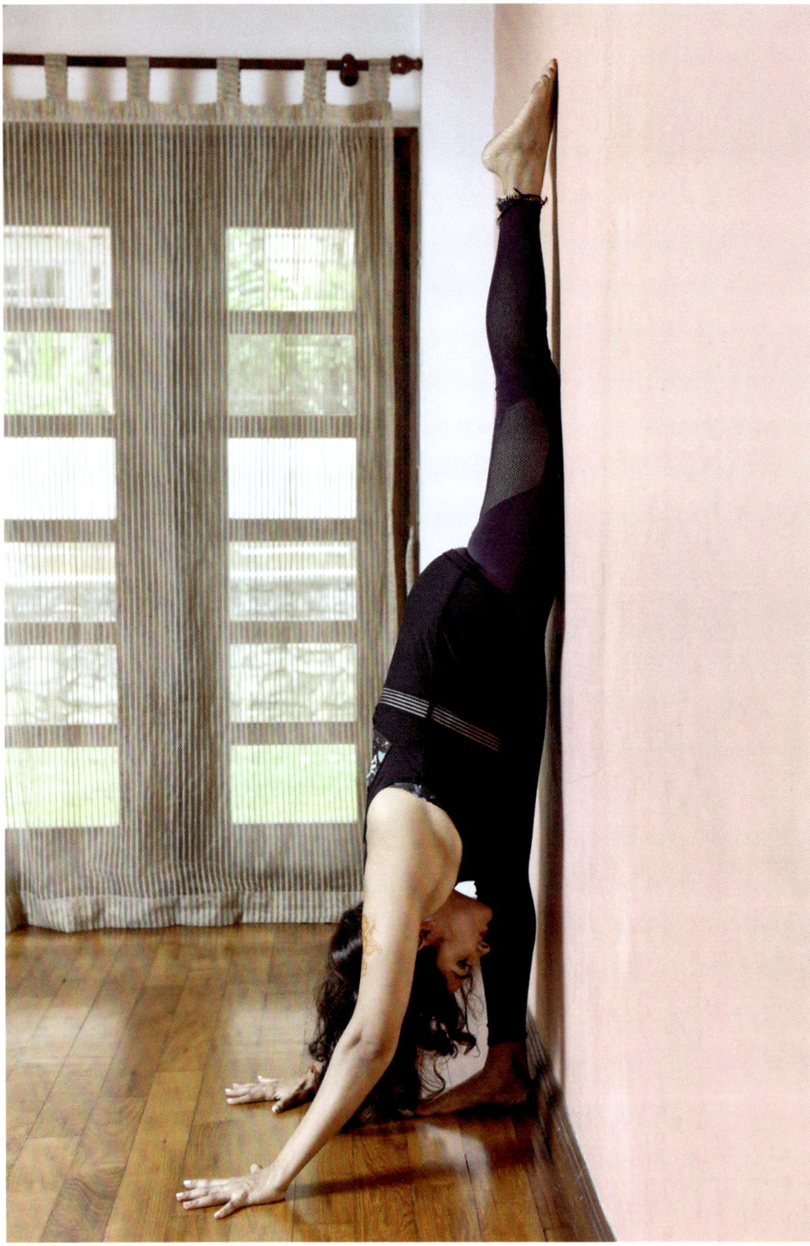

Artistic Pose: Inverted Wall *Hanumanasana*

Life as a Vinyasa

Our lives can be seen through the lens of a yoga practice as a vinyasa: a sequential flow from asana to asana as we move from experience to experience. The direction, as we go through each experience, is to keep our minds open to learning and our hearts open to love.

Patanjali laid down specific paths to establish a strong yoga practice. As our practice deepens, our minds attune to each of them so deeply that they simply become the way we live.

Tapah svadhyaya isvarapranidhanani kriya yogah
Tapas *(intense effort)*, svadhyaya *(self-study and reflection on one's own self)* and isvarapranidhanani *(surrender to God) constitute the yoga of kriya (action).*[1]

Patanjali's *Yoga Sutras*, chapter 2, sutra 1

Each of these elements is vital in the progress of a yoga practitioner. In the very first verse of the first chapter, yoga is described as

1 'Manasa Yoga' *Teacher Training Notes.*

shasanam, a discipline. While growing up, the word discipline was anathema to me. But as I grew up, I realized that nothing meaningful could be realized without discipline. To achieve excellence in any field, be it academics, sports, work, business or yoga practice, burning hard effort or *tapas*, is essential. Guruji B.K.S. Iyengar himself practiced yoga for a phenomenal number of hours a day, every day of his life. You have to allow the zeal of your purpose to consume you as you strive for excellence in your chosen path.

There is no substitute for consistent practice. My own asana practice has grown tremendously over the years, and it brings me the greatest satisfaction that, with the passing of time, my body is actually stronger and more flexible than it has ever been before. When I began my meditative sitting practices, like most raw beginners, I too was consumed by doubt. What was I doing? Was I doing it right? Is there was any point to this? Should I watch my breath, or chant a mantra, or count, or do it all? But something within myself told me that this was the path for me, and so I held on tight despite all my doubts and questions. With consistent practice, the flavour of my meditative practices also changed. The restlessness and questions that plagued me gave way to a genuine desire to have quiet time to myself. I began to truly cherish the time, and this joy inspired me to consciously create it. In times of intense trauma, it became my lifeline, a space where I could come face-to-face with the sadness and grief that consumed my mind, release it and start my day with renewed faith and guidance. Now even on holidays I actively create time and space to meditate wherever I am—on the beach to the sound of the waves, or while my mind gets absorbed in the breathtaking artistic display of colours splashed across the sky as the sun sets on the distant horizon.

Effort and Restraint

While in one sense *tapas* can be taken as a commitment and dedication to intense practice, it can also be a principle to release ourselves from situations that don't honour us and patterns that debilitate us. So while *tapas* is in the doing, it is also in the non-doing, in the abstinence, in the holding back. The ethic of *tapas* has to become a way of life, integrated into every fiber of our being. It has to become the way we work and approach every situation in our lives. It is only then that excellence becomes our way of life.

Tapas is referred to as 'burning effort' and thus has a refining quality to it. The more you heat gold, the more purified it becomes. So the fire of *tapas* burns away the impurities of our minds and bodies—our sloth, laziness, procrastination tendencies, restless energies, our clinging and attachment patterns. Through *tapas*, we connect to our own inner power and strength, become single-minded in our focus, and dedicated to our path.

Svadhyaya or self-study is another vital element of yoga practice. In fact, I believe that the whole of life, from birth to death offers us an opportunity to practice *svadhyaya*. The only problem is that from birth we are unconsciously trained to look outward and learn about everything outside of ourselves! As kids we are taught numbers and the alphabet, and then comes science, history and geography. As we continue to study, we follow our interests and maybe learn about cars or the solar system or buildings. Or maybe we pursue our interest in food, fashion or design. But nowhere are we directed to learn about ourselves!

It is only if we are naturally inclined that we start studying ourselves from an early age or, if we are fortunate, through the hard knocks of life, we get shoved out of our comfort zones and forced to confront our inner demons and struggles. But whatever the manner that brings us to this path, it is a lifelong journey to greater understanding, clarity, and wisdom—to evolving into our highest selves.

As we study ourselves and the dark areas of our lives where we suffer, we are forced to confront our deep attachments, our possessive tendencies, our demands and conditions, the situations where we cling and hold on despite seeing the writing on the wall, our inability to release addictive patterns of eating and lifestyle that rob us of good health and sometimes life itself. Do we take responsibility for the state of our lives and our minds? Or do we just go through life assigning blame to everybody else around us? Are we defensive and do we make excuses every single time we are pulled up? Initially, we may be unable to do very much, except simply observe. But with continuous seeing and understanding, eventually wisdom dawns, and we draw on reserves of courage that we never knew we had to take action that is right by us. We begin to own our power.

While *tapas* and *svadhyaya* are very necessary along the path of yoga, it is also important to be aligned to the concept of *isvara pranidhana,* or surrender to God. Life is never smooth. It throws us bends and curves when we least expect it. That is the beauty and the heartbreak of life, the proverbial agony and ecstasy.

Some of the most beautiful people I know have gone through the most intense suffering. One of my aunts spent the last 20 years of her life selflessly taking care of her unmarried siblings; nursing them herself single-handedly through old age and ill health until they passed away. In her lifetime, she also had to deal with the unimaginable grief of losing not one, but two of her sons. But surrendering to the verses from the Gita is her refuge and her strength. Some of the most amazing and philanthropic men that I have had the privilege of knowing closely, who have truly made a difference in hundreds of lives and lived meaningful purposeful lives themselves, have had to go through periods of intense suffering in the last days of their lives. Another beautiful friend I have has to deal with the diagnosis of a progressive neurological disease that has restricted her life at a physical level. Some students struggle with infertility, while some others have suffered two or three miscarriages.

Life is not math. One plus one is never two. We could have all the formulae for happiness, we could follow the rules to the T, but it does not guarantee anything. There is a strange working to the universe—a method to the seeming madness that is beyond the comprehension of the normal parameters of the human mind. Thus, the concept of *isvara pranidhana* becomes all the more relevant. It is an awareness and surrender to the knowing that there is a broader perspective to the universe that our limited minds are unable to rationally comprehend. That what is asked of us at all points is to put in our intense effort, continue on the path of studying, exploring and understanding ourselves, and ultimately, dedicate and surrender the fruits of our efforts to the unknown workings of the universe, to *isvara*.

This profound attitude, absorbed and cultivated as a philosophy, will anchor us, especially in times of great distress—when logic and reason fail, when we cannot make sense of events and situations that arise, when people we trusted with our lives walk away, when all our hard work and dedication does not bring the results we envisaged on the job front, when we get stricken by a terminal illness, when people we love die young. When life brings us to our knees, when in sheer desperation we throw off the bowlines and set sail into the vast unknown, then the concept of *isvara pranidhana* is the wind on our backs.

This resonates very closely with one of the most famous verses of the Bhagavad Gita, chapter 2, verse 47:

Karmanye Vadhikaraste Ma Phaleshu Kadachana, Ma Karmaphalaheturbhurma Te Sangostvakarmani

You have the right (adhikara) *to work* (karma) *only but never* (kadachana) *to its fruits* (phala). *Let not* (ma) *the fruits of action* (karmaphala) *be your motive* (hetu), *nor let your attachment* (sanaga) *be to inaction* (akarmanai).[2]

The benevolence of surrender is that it takes our minds into a state of acceptance. All suffering comes from resistance. The more we resist, the more we suffer. But when we view challenging situations through the lens of surrender, especially when we have given it our best and there is nothing else we can do, it becomes easier for us to accept that which we cannot control—another person's actions and emotions towards us, specific situations on the job front, our children's interests and their right to lead their lives the best way they see fit, illnesses that afflict us despite our best efforts to stay fit and eat right. What we can do is see the learning opportunity in each experience, strive for equanimity in the face of our misfortune, and evolve stronger, wiser and more compassionate from the whole process.

There is no end to education. It is not that you read a book, pass an examination and finish with education. The whole of life, from the moment you are born to the moment you die, is a process of learning.[3]

—Jiddu Krishnamurti

2 Paramahansa Yogananda, *God Talks with Arjuna: The Bhagavad Gita* (Kolkata: Yagoda Satsanga Society of India, 2011).

3 Jiddu Krishnamurti, *Krishnamurti on Education* (Chennai: Krishnamurti Foundation India, 2003).

Like a flowing stream of water, we too have to develop the ability to let go and flow where the sometimes-rocky currents of life take us, as we can't ever swim against it. So instead of kicking, screaming and railing against the unfairness of life, why not surrender in grace and flow in acceptance in a larger universal plan? It will not happen overnight but it's the only direction that's worth pursuing.

Let Your Light Blaze

We all have light within us. But why is it that some people seem to stand taller, shine brighter than others? The example that I use, which can be easily understood, is that of a filament in a light bulb. The light emitting from the filament is the same. But if the bulb that surrounds it is covered with dust or dirt, then the light that shines through is dimmed. On the contrary, if the bulb is clean and transparent then the light from the filament shines brightly.

So it is with us. We have to meticulously clean the dirt and grime off the surface of the mind (read: bulb)—the judgment, the conditioning, the demands, the possessiveness, the clinging, the ignorance, the misapprehension, the envy, the jealousy, and the fear. We have to be aware and accept the state of our lives, the circumstances that we find ourselves in, the patterns of our mind, and know that they are the breeding ground of these emotions that block our inherent radiance. Through awareness, through self-study, through the practice of the various limbs of yoga, as we release the negativities in ourselves bit-by-bit, the divine inner light reflects in our personality and our relationships as love, friendliness, respect, compassion, equanimity, non-violence, non-judgment, openness, flexibility, truthfulness, appreciation and contentment.

The more we accept where we are now, the less turbulent our minds are, and the more connected we are to our inner selves, our power and our light.

It reminds me of the sacred Gayatri Mantra,

Om bhur bhuvah suvah
Tat savitur varenyam
bhargo devasya dhimahi
dhiyo yonah prachodayat

Om bhur bhuvah suvah - bhur refers to the earth plane, which we link to as the world of physicality, *bhuvah* refers to the mind plane with all the thoughts and emotions, and *suvah* in the Manasa system refers to the plane of subtler *samskaras* or seed patterns of our being in an unexpressed state. So everything we know and don't know about ourselves is represented by Om.

Tat savitur varenyam bhargo devasya dhimahi - 'tat' refers to 'that', which here is symbolically represented as the *savitah* or the sun. The sun stands for light, which, in the context of yoga, is the light of awareness. That light which is radiant with *bhargah*—the effulgence of wisdom, to that light we offer our *dhimahi*—intellect.

Dhiyo yo nah prachodayat - And as we offer our *dhi* or intellect, *dhiyah*, may that great light, *yo*, direct and inspire our ways of thinking towards our own highest possibilities.

Practice

1. ***Tapas***: Set out a general plan for your day or week. Time for asana practice, time for sitting practice, reading scriptures, contemplating them etc., and try and stick to it.
2. ***Svadhyaya***: Journal about your day every night before you go to bed. Use it as an opportunity to review your day, see where

you responded well, and where you could have done better. Through the meticulous approach of self-study, we can slowly refine ourselves; releasing patterns that don't serve us, and focusing on those that do.

3. ***Isvara pranidhana:*** Cultivate an attitude of surrender. The more we know, the more we realize we don't know. What is the energy that causes my fingers to type, your eyes to read, your mind to comprehend, your breath to flow? Slowly a sense that 'I am not the doer' develops and we are able to release our need for 'control' and accept the way life flows towards us.

Asanas: *Isvara pranidhana* - Surrender Through Forward Bends

While the invitation of life is to evolve into our highest possibilities, sometimes situations challenge and shake us to our very core. When there are no answers, when we cannot understand with our rational logical mind, we surrender to the wisdom of the infinite universal intelligence and we embody that in our asana practice through forward bends.

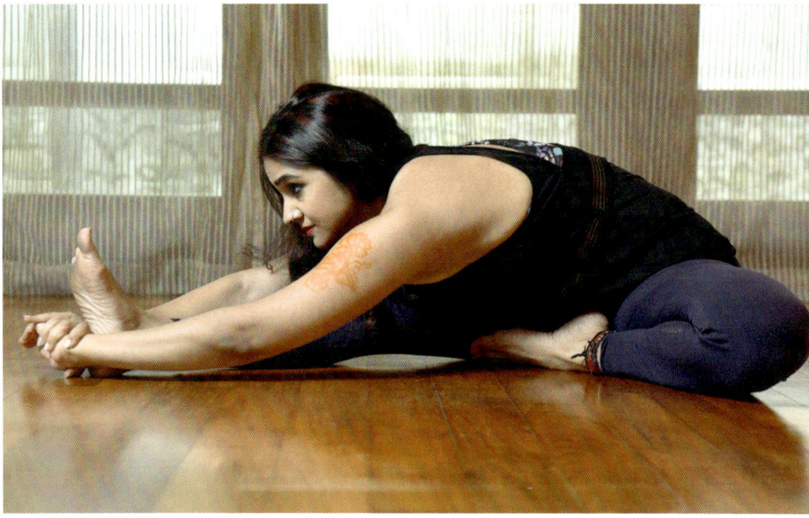

Janushirsasana: Seated One-Leg Forward Bend

1. Sit with your legs extended out in front of you.
2. Externally rotate your right leg and bend your right knee, bringing your right heel towards the pubis. Press the sole of your right foot against your left inner thigh.
3. Press your left hand onto the floor on the left side, and gently twist your pelvis and torso, so that your navel points towards the direction of your left foot.
4. As you inhale, lift your right arm up, and as you exhale, extend forward through the right side of your torso and your arm so that your chest extends over your left thigh. Clasp your shin, your foot or a strap looped over your foot.
5. Then take your left hand forward and clasp with both hands. Make sure your left elbow crease does not get in front of your right elbow crease.

Stay for 5–10 breaths. Inhale and lift your arms up. Exhale and release. Change legs and repeat on the other side.

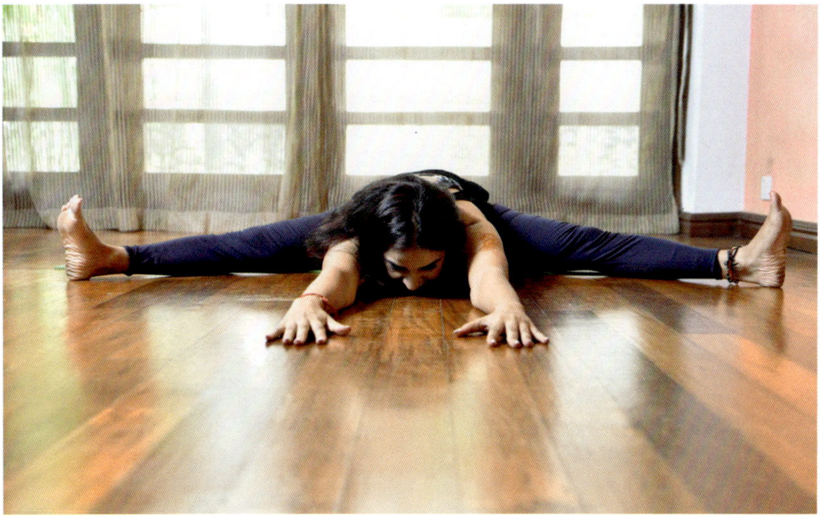

Upavistakonasana: Seated Wide-Leg Forward Fold

1. Sit on the mat with your legs spread out as wide as possible.
2. Keep your legs straight and active. Make sure your toes are pointing upward.
3. Shift to the front edge of the sit bones by pressing down through the inner edges of your heels.
4. Pressing the buttocks backward, extend further forward from your hips, with your hands on the floor.
5. With each inhale, extend the heart forward, and move your hands a few steps forward. With each exhale, relax carefully towards the floor. Remember, rather than moving your head to the floor, think about keeping your chest to the floor.

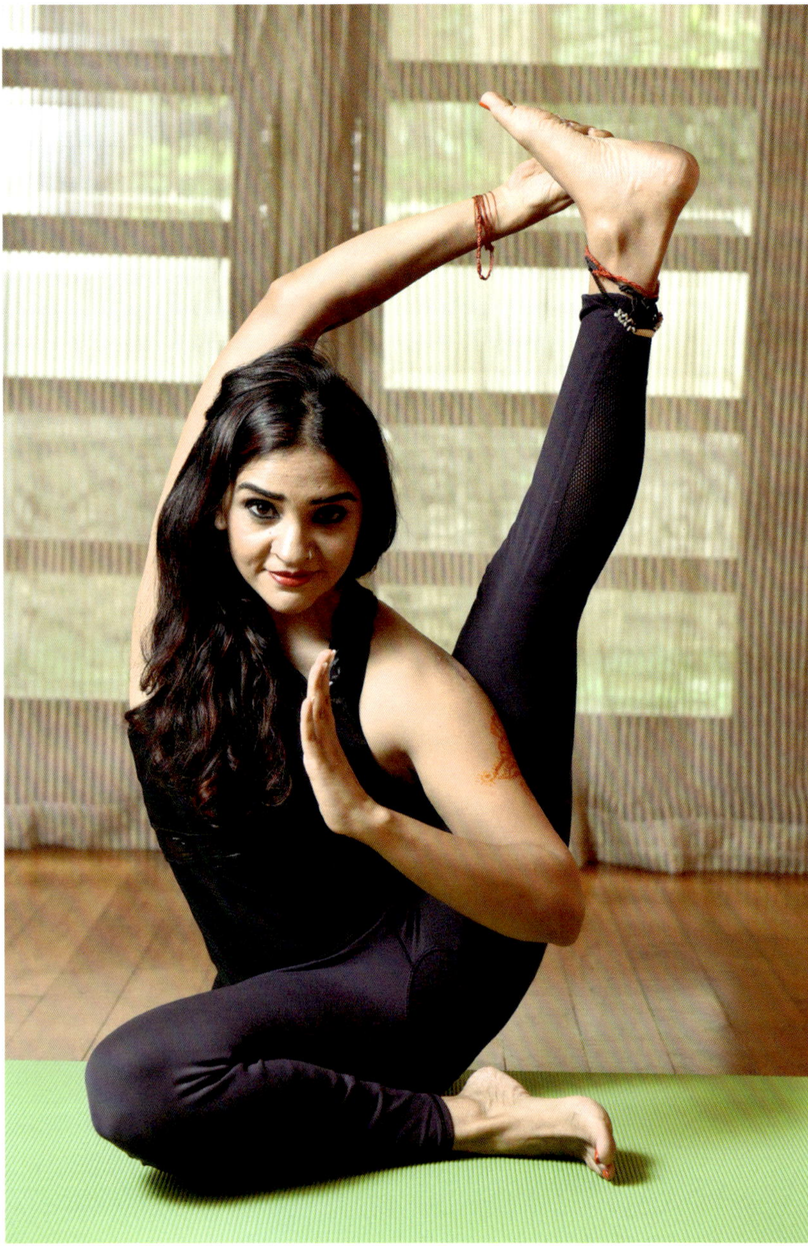

Artistic Pose: *Urdhvaparsva Janusirsasana*

Follow Your Bliss

The success of yoga does not lie in the ability to perform postures but in how it positively changes the way we live our life and our relationships.[1]

—T.K.V. Desikachar

Growing up, I had led a very sheltered life with very little exposure. Even though I grew up in Coimbatore, India, yoga was never even in the periphery of my life! Only one of my uncles, a cardiologist who lived in the US, practiced yoga regularly. He had a short temper, and had been diagnosed with a heart condition early on. So he consciously embarked on a regular practice of asana and meditation. I vividly recall one scene where we were at the airport and his flight was delayed. Instead of getting mad and losing his temper like he otherwise would have, I saw him sit by himself in a chair, close his eyes and focus on his breath! It left an impression on me early on at how much yoga practice helped his temperament and physical well-being.

1 T.K.V. Desikachar and R.H. Cravens, *Health, Healing and Beyond: Yoga and the Living Tradition of T. Krishnamacharya* (New York: North Point Press, 2011).

Today, three cardiac bypass surgeries later at the age of eighty, he is still going strong and is still very enthusiastic about his yoga practice. I have no doubt that it is his committed yoga practice that has sustained him well over the years.

As an adult, for many years I struggled with 'my path' and did some intense soul-searching about the purpose of my life. Yoga was just something I did because it helped and healed me. At a point in my life when I was disturbed, restless and searching for a better way to live, I instinctively sought refuge in yoga practice. That gradually led to a desire to share what had helped my own life with others. Thus, the pursuit of teaching yoga, and the subsequent setting up of my yoga studio about five years ago.

When I first moved to Malaysia in 1997 after my marriage, it presented me with the opportunity to start afresh. When I thought about work, I realised that the only job that brought me joy and satisfaction was writing, and that led me to apply for my first job as a writer. Though that job lasted only six months, it set me up as a freelance writer. I worked with leading women's magazines as a writer and columnist, writing mostly on health, parenting, yoga and fitness.

Later, in 1999, yoga came into my life. Mataji Divyananda, who at that point managed the Integral Yoga Institute in Coimbatore, India, inspired me to take up the practice. The next year, when I came back, she encouraged me to pursue a teacher-training program, which I did, and began teaching soon after. When I came back to Malaysia, I was guided to Manoj Kaimal. From the very first class I was inspired by Manoj's teachings, where every asana was backed with precise anatomical instructions weaved together with in-depth yogic philosophy, including *sankhya*, sutras, vedanta and tantra. This made each class a truly transformative experience. I knew right away that this is how I wanted to teach too and meaningfully impact my students, not just at a physical level, in terms of how to create the shape of an asana, but in a way that profoundly affected their states of mind and their lives.

In the meantime I continued freelancing as a yoga teacher as well, as it seemed most convenient with a young child and a husband who was always traveling. But freelancing was not very fulfilling. It lacked the satisfaction that comes with having students who connected and evolved with me over a period of time. So as soon as my second son Krishan started school, I set up my own yoga studio, 'Mat and Beyond Yoga Studio'.

Follow Your Bliss

The reason I am sharing all this is just to say that at every point in my life, I have simply 'followed my bliss'. After having made costly mistakes in my youth, I figured out early on that life was too short to do anything else. And if today I have satisfaction and fulfilment in my life as a yoga teacher, writer and speaker, it is only because of this one maxim. It also gave me the greatest gift of all, the ability to touch the lives of my students positively and make a difference through my classes and my words.

Samahita Chitta

In order to connect to our inner self, what is important is that our minds are in the state of *samahita chitta*—an evenly-settled state of consciousness. If our minds are constantly agitated, restless and reactive (*vyutthana chitta*), we get caught up at a surface level in the restless agitated chatter of the mind, and are unable to sink deep. It is impossible to gain insights or to experience states of boundless awareness in these reactive states. That can happen only if the mind is calm and tranquil over a period of time with *sattva*, the dominant taste of consciousness.

Thus the practice of the different limbs of the Ashatanga yoga as set out by Patanjali: *Yamas* (ethical practices), *Niyamas* (observances), Asana (postures), Pranayama (breathing practices), Pratyahara (withdrawal of the senses), *Dharana* (concentration) and Dhyana (meditation) serves to evoke a tranquil and settled state of consciousness in the practitioner.

Yogaanganusthanath ashuddhiksaye jnanadiptih avivekakhyateh
By being established in the practice (anusthanath) *of the different limbs of yoga* (yogaanga) *impurities* (ashuddhi) *weaken* (ksaye) *light of wisdom radiates* (jnanadiptih) *leading to discriminative discernment* (avivekakhyateh)[2]

—Patanjali's *Yoga Sutras*, chapter 2, sutra 28

Patanjali also offers *parikarman* (methods of purifying the consciousness) in the form of attitudes that we could cultivate in chapter 1, sutra 33 to achieve that state of *chitta prasadanam* (favorably disposed, benevolent disposition of consciousness). Swami Satchidananda, in his book *The Yoga Sutras of Patanjali* says '*Whether you are interested in reaching* samadhi *or plan to ignore yoga entirely, I would advise you to remember this one sutra*'. He also adds, '*In my own experience, this sutra became my guiding light to keep my mind serene always*'.[3]

Maître karuna mudita upekshanam sukha dukha punya a-punya vishayanam bhavanatash chitta prasadanam
By cultivating the sentiments of friendship towards those who are happy; compassion towards those who are suffering, goodwill towards those

2 'Manasa Yoga' *Teacher Training Notes.*

3 Swami Satchidananda, trans., *The Yoga Sutras of Patanjali* (USA: Integral Yoga Publications, 2004).

who are virtuous and indifference towards those the non-virtuous, the consciousness is purified and made pleasant.[4]

—Patanjali's *Yoga Sutras*, chapter 1, sutra 33

Know Your Gunas

Consciousness or *chitta* is composed of the three attributes of nature: rajas, tamas and sattva. Each attribute has its own distinct characteristics. Every human being is composed of all three gunas. It is the variation in the proportion of the three gunas that accounts for the heterogeneous variety of human beings.

Rajas: Rajas is aggression, energy, activity, ambition, restlessness and passion. A person who is more 'rajasic' in nature is a whirlwind of activity and involved with the affairs of the world.

Tamas: Tamas is characterized by a state of inertia, dullness, lethargy, laziness, and darkness to name a few. A person steeped in tamas leads a dull and inactive life.

Sattva: Illumination, reflection, purity, nobility, responsibility and calm are some words that characterize sattva. A person whose state of consciousness is predominantly 'satvic' is poised, mature, contemplative and equipoised.

Our direction in yoga practice and in life is to increase the sattva content in our consciousness, manage the energy of rajas and reduce tamas correspondingly.

Express Your Light

This is the tag line of my studio and it beautifully sums up the inspiration to take up the practice of yoga—to express our light!

4 Manoj Kaimal, *Making Patanjali Palatable* (Manoj Kaimal, 2008).

The more receptive and stable our minds are, the more we are able to connect to our inner self—to what moves us, what inspires us, what makes us happy, what motivates us, and what triggers our unhappiness. Over a period of time this sensitizes us to the subtlest movements of the universal force, shakti, that flows through us. The more attuned we are to this force, the more we are able to express it through our creativity.

For some of us this can be expressed through our words as writers, for some others it's through art, paintings and designing, and for yet some others it is through music or dance. It could be expressed through yoga sequences that we constantly create as yoga teachers, through dance sequences, in the recipes that we churn up every day as we cook for our families, or in exploring new ways to exercise our bodies! Whatever the channel and manner in which the creative force chooses to express itself through us, connecting to the flow of this force, through our creativity, is truly a gift and a grace, and expressing it is our innate responsibility, one that yields immeasurable joy and fulfillment.

Creativity is the throb and heartbeat of life. As we consciously harness it in our lives, the joy and satisfaction we experience in its expression is matchless and endless, as the universal force Shakti, herself, is dynamic and limitless.

We can consciously cultivate and strengthen our connection to this universal energy, to the vast field of potentiality that lies within us—by going inwards, and through spending some time in meditation and silence every day. When we express ourselves from that space, it lends a purity and depth to all our creative endeavours. The more we tap into it, the more it reveals itself to us. The more we express it, the greater our attunement and flow of inspiration.

Connect to who you truly are—what grips you, what moves you, what brings you joy, what your strengths are, regardless of whether it is being a dumpling kicker, a cookie eater, a dancer, or someone who just likes to hug (from the movie 'Kung Fu Panda 4'). Be gloriously proud of each role and identity you are called to play and express it to your fullest. *Svabittau kalayati,* a phrase from the ancient scripture *Spanda Karikas*, states that the ONE light refracts itself out as myriad of resplendent unique lights (each one of us). So CELEBRATE YOU!

As our connection with our inner self deepens, as our awareness and consciousness expands, it leads to greater clarity, wisdom and understanding. We see the world and interact in our relationships with greater openness, sensitivity and a broader perspective.

Most importantly, we own our power. We become less reliant on validation from the outside world;—from peers, partners, bosses etc. We become less dependent on relationships to inspire and motivate us to our highest selves, and we become less seeking and take responsibility for our own salvation.

Through silence and meditation, we are guided by the intelligence that flows through all of us. We receive validation and joy from the satisfaction and fulfilment that comes from expressing ourselves through our creative endeavours. Through our efforts and the benevolence of grace, we strengthen our connection to our inner selves, which reflects in love, respect and compassion for ourselves and others.

Yoga chitta vritti nirodha

Yoga is the nirodha, *dissolution of* vritti, *fluctuations in the* chitta, *consciousness.*[5]

—Patanjali's *Yoga Sutras,* chapter 1, sutra 2

5 Manoj Kaimal, *Making Patanjali Palatable* (Manoj Kaimal, 2008).

So why do we practice yoga? The answer is revealed in this sutra. *Chitta* or consciousness includes the mind, ego and intellect, and this is where we face all problems—feeling disrespected and unvalued, feelings of anxiety, fear, restlessness, agitation and confusion. Through the practice of the Ashtanga yoga (the eight limbs of yoga), the confusion and the disturbances lessen, the mind settles and we get a taste of our essential nature.

The Mind and the Ocean

The mind is likened to an ocean. Like the surface of the ocean is choppy, similarly, the surface level of the mind too, in its natural unconscious state, is disturbed and restless. So we generally connect with feelings of frustration, impatience, agitation, etc. But as the surface of the ocean settles, when we look, we can get a clear reflection of ourselves. Similarly, through reflective, contemplative and meditative practices, as the waves of the mind become still, we are able to connect to that deeper essence of ourselves rather than the surface that we generally identify with.

With consistent meditative practice, we can attune and practice being present to the moment as it unfolds—to the person having a conversation with us, to the task at hand, or to the sunset in front of us. As our minds become less turbulent and reactive, we become more attuned to our inner world. We connect to inspiration, to flashes of insight, to a quiet intuitive knowing, to a flow of words, to guidance that comes to us from conversations we have, to a deep understanding of ourselves and our paths. Confusion gives way to clarity, ignorance is replaced with surety, and diffidence bows over to self-esteem and confidence. Universal timing comes into play through synchronicities and, like the threads of a fabric, divine orchestration ensures that seemingly random occurrences are woven into a well-lit path.

As the verse from the ancient philosophical and yogic texts, the Puranas goes:

Yat Pinde, Tat Brahmande
What is there in the microcosm is also there in the macrocosm. As is the body, so is the universe. All separation is an illusion.
So as we find ourselves, we find the universe too.

Practice

1. Be conscious of how you feel. Be aware of what energizes you, brings you joy, leaves you feeling elated and exhilarated, boosts your self-esteem. Do that as often as you can.
2. As you turn inward, you will sense naturally what creative pursuit brings you joy. For some it may be writing children's stories, for some others it maybe composing lyrics to music or cooking creatively, and yet for others it is expressing their inner resonance with easels and paints. Connect to the subtle movements of the mind and emotions. They hold the key to understanding yourself better.
3. Do this regularly. Doing anything becomes effortless when you revel in the joy, in the doing of it. Express it. The more we express our creative gift, the greater is our attunement and stronger the flow of inspiration.
4. Be sensitive to the world—to the learning that is all around, to the guidance that the universe is imparting to you. Over a period of time you begin to understand its language, teaching and direction.

Asanas: Lateral Flow

Life is about living in the flow! Allow the creative force to flow through you in this series of lateral asanas.

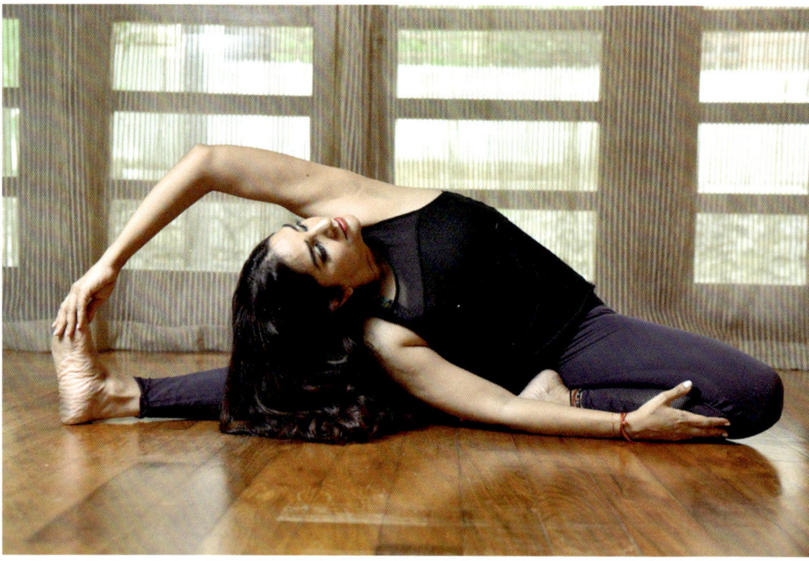

Parivritta Janushirsasana

1. Sit with your legs straight in front of you.
2. Bend your right leg, shift your right buttock back, and take your right heel towards the root of your right thigh. Your chest should be parallel to a wall on your right side, so that you are in a lateral orientation to your left leg.
3. Inhale, and as you exhale, laterally tilt your pelvis to the left and lower your left elbow towards the floor, inside of your left leg. If your elbow does not reach the floor, place a block or pillow for your left elbow and forearm to rest on.
4. Take your right arm overhead, and reach towards your left foot. Initially you might not be able to clasp your foot, and you can use a strap on your left foot to hold. Keep rotating the front of your rib cage upward, away from your left inner thigh.

Stay for 5–10 breaths. Inhale as you come back up, and repeat on the other side.

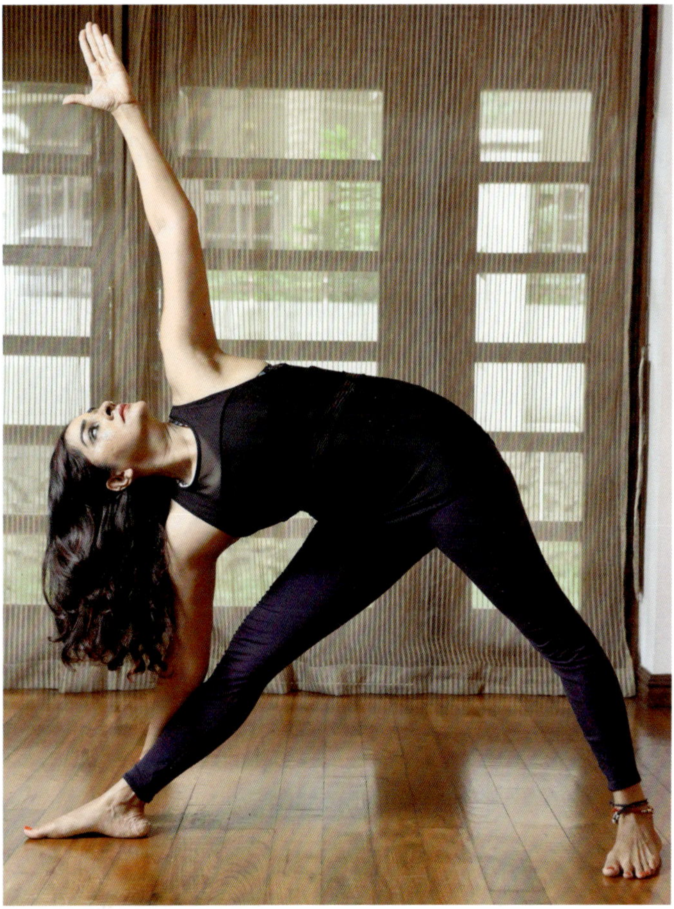

Trikonasana: Triangle

1. Stand with your feet wide apart. Inhale and lift your arms up to shoulder height.
2. Exhale and turn your right leg to the right. Laterally tilt your hip to the right, extend your right arm to the right, and then lower your hand towards the floor. You may place your hand on your shin, a block, or on the floor.
3. Rotate the front of your rib cage towards the ceiling and lift your left arm up towards the ceiling.

Hold for 5–10 breaths. Inhale, rise up and repeat on the other side.

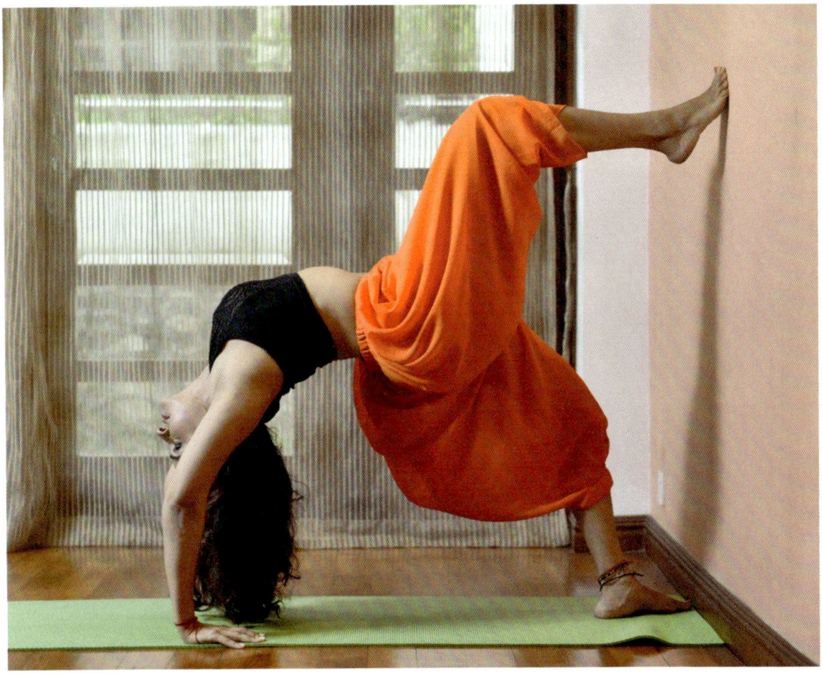

Artistic Picture: *Ekapada Urdhva Dhanurasana*

Why Should We Practice Yoga?

Spirituality is not some external goal that one must seek, but a part of the divine core of each of us, which we must reveal.[1]

—Guruji B.K.S. Iyengar

As a teacher I get many questions from students, the most common among them being—can yoga help me lose weight? Can I reduce stress? Will it help my back pain? Will it help my relationships? Will it bring my family together? There are also many questions regarding lifestyle—do I have to become vegetarian? Do I have to give up sugar or eat organic? Will I become an environmental activist?

Let me share what I have discovered. Years of consistent yoga practice brings a consciousness, a sensitivity, to our relationship with ourselves—our physical, mental, emotional and spiritual states, and to our relationship with the world around us. We become more conscious of what we are eating, what we are thinking, what

1 B.K.S. Iyengar, *Light on Life: The Yoga Journey to Wholesomeness, Inner Peace, and Ultimate Freedom*, (USA: Rodale Inc., 2005).

our intentions are, what we are talking about, to who we are speaking, our exercise and lifestyle patterns, our emotions and the way we feel, the manner in which we react, our ability or inability to focus due to our incessant need to check our phones out of sheer restlessness or as an addictive pattern, our ability or inability to respond appropriately, the fact that we are engaging with someone out of boredom and not because it particularly stimulates us, our energy levels at different points during the day, our energy levels before and after conversations with different people, in different situations. We begin to naturally become conscious of it all.

And as we become conscious, we begin to take responsibility for the state of our lives too, as we cannot take cover beneath the shield of unconsciousness anymore. A clarity arises about our roles in the different experiences that manifest in our lives. For example, if we become obese or pre-diabetic, instead of only blaming our genes, maybe we could cut down on sugar and work on getting regular exercise. When we hear ourselves always complaining about lack of time, we become aware of time spent mindlessly watching junk television or browsing through other people's profiles on Facebook. In this manner, we regain our power to create the body, health and life that we seek, instead of blaming external circumstances for our current state of affairs.

'To be human is to be conscious—the only issue is how conscious. For the mind, awareness is the womb of creation. To achieve a life filled with meaning, you must figure out how to be more conscious; only then do you become the author of your own destiny.' [2]

—Deepak Chopra and Rudolph E. Tanzi

2 Deepak Chopra and Rudolph E. Tanzi, *Super Brain: Unleashing the Explosive Power of Your Mind to Maximize Health, Happiness, and Spiritual Well-Being* (London: Rider Books, 2011).

Create Our Lives

This practice also connects us with the important capacity of choosing our point of focus. Most of our life we are led by our wayward monkey minds. The mind get happy or sad, fills with rage or peace, alternates between bouts of depression and exultation, and we think that is the only way to live, at the mercy of our minds. But through yoga practice, as we begin to take baby steps towards consciously directing our minds—bringing awareness to our feet, our sit bones, our spine, watching and counting our breath etc., we step into the process of working with the mind—channeling it, directing it, holding our attention. And we practice this in the neutral, non-aggressive atmosphere of a yoga class, which is most conducive to allowing this 'mental work'.

With regular practice, we become adept in working with our minds and, by strengthening our capacity to shift our point of focus, we ultimately own our power to shift our states of minds and, thus, our lives.

We develop the ability to see our inner narrative and exercise our faculty of choice to tweak our mindscape by consciously changing our perspective to view any experience as necessary to the learning, evolving, and individuation process. As we become more conscious, we are able to be creatively reborn on a moment-to-moment basis.

All the tenets of yoga encapsulated in the *yamas* (restraints) of Ashtanga yoga as laid out by Patanjali—ahimsa (non-violence), *satya* (truth), *asteya* (non-stealing), *aparigraha* (non grasping), *brahmacharya* (seeing Brahman in everything), can be practiced in asana by expressing the intentions of love, respect, compassion and truth towards our bodies and then towards the outside world. In class, we honour the unique journeys that our bodies have been through, from brain surgery, spine surgery and arthritis to back problems and wrist injuries, by respecting that in yoga practice and not causing further himsa (violence) towards ourselves at a physical or mental level. So, if we are suffering from back pain, even if our neighbor is doing 10 drop-backs continuously, we maintain *upekshanam*, our equanimity, and remain respectful of our backs without our minds plunging into self-criticism or worse, actually attempting it and causing more violence to the body in the process!

The conscious work is to shift the mind to focus on what you can do! The transformation and evolution to be the best version of ourselves—kinder, compassionate, loving, equanimous, less judgmental, conditional and goal oriented—begins right there on the mat, and we take that with us to meet the everyday challenges and situations that arise in our lives. While it is great to read scriptures and recite mantras, the ultimate test is to live it, for that is how it will reflect in our thoughts, words, actions and relationships.

> *The source of my father's teaching, and the essence of Yoga, was formulated by the great Indian sage, Patanjali, more than two thousand years ago in this succinct definition: Yoga is the ability to direct the mind exclusively toward an object and sustain that direction without any distractions. That object can be something as concrete as a work of art, as dynamic as a runner's race, or as abstract as a mathematical formula. It can be as personal and internal to an individual as an exploration of the question 'Who am I?' Or it can be as transcendent as being 'one with the Lord' whether conceived as a named God or a nameless truth.*[3]
>
> —T.K.V. Desikachar

3 T.K.V. Desikachar and R.H. Cravens, *Health, Healing, and Beyond: Yoga and the Living Tradition of T. Krishnamacharya* (New York: North Point Press, 2011).

In this manner, by doing the inner work, by owning our power, everything that we desire—from inner peace, a healthy body weight, and a strong flexible body, to becoming a conscious consumer or even a green activist—is ours for the taking. But know that it is a continuously-unfolding process, a practice that must be pursued over *dirgha kala* (long period of time), *nairantarya* (continuously), *satkara* (with respect) and *asevita* (with complete observance) in order to be *dridha bhumi* (firmly established).

Sa tu dirgha kala nairantarya satkarasevito drdha bhumih
The practice is said to have laid a firm foundation only after being pursued with total commitment, and for a long time without interruption.[4]

—Patanjali's *Yoga Sutras*, chapter 1, verse 14

Asana practice is, for me, living spirituality. The practice takes us first into the expressed form that each one of us is used to in an individualized manner. But as our awareness deepens in the asana, we start to recognize the formless infinite intelligence of the universe coalescing with the form of the body. Then we resonate with the words of Guruji B.K.S. Iyengar; '*The body is my temple, asanas are my prayers*'. In his book *Light on Life* he says:

> *What I teach is spiritual practice in action. I use the body to discipline the mind and to reach the soul. Asanas, when done with the right intention, will help to transform an individual by taking the person away from an awareness of just the body towards the consciousness of the soul. Indeed, as I often say, body is the bow, asana the arrow, and soul is the target.*[5]

4 Manoj Kaimal, *Making Patanjali Palatable* (Manoj Kaimal, 2008).

5 B.K.S. Iyengar, *Light on Life: The Yoga Journey to Wholesomeness, Inner Peace, and Ultimate Freedom,* (USA: Rodale Inc., 2005).

In the words of Swami Satchidananda, from his book *Beyond Words*, '*You are all sparks of the divinity, images of God. You are nothing less than God himself. You have that divinity, that goodness, that peace, and that perfect health. That is your true nature, so why should you run after anything?*'[6]

One of my favourite inspiring phrases oft repeated by my teacher, Manoj Kaimal, and derived from the scripture *Spanda Karikas* is:

You are Spanda of Shankara, a resplendent spark of Shankara

So keep the faith, live the practice, enjoy the journey and allow for the magic to manifest in your life. Express your divine light! Celebrate life!

I end with the invocation of the powerful universal Shanti Mantra for peace:

Sarvesham Svastir Bhavatu; May good health be unto all
Sarvesham Shantir Bhavatu; May peace be unto all
Sarvesham Purnam Bhavatu; May fullness be unto all
Sarvesham Mangalam Bhavatu; May auspiciousness be unto all
Om Shanti Shanti Shanti

---

6 Swami Satchidananda, *Beyond Words* (Toronto: Holt, Rinehart and Winston of Canada, Limited, 1977).

References

Books

Bhagwan Shree Rajneesh. 1989. *The Sword and the Lotus.* Ed. Ma Dhyan Sagar. Köln, Germany: Rebel Publishing House.

Byron, Thomas. 2012. *The Dhammapada: The Sayings of the Buddha.* New York: Vintage Books.

Chopra, Deepak and Rudolph E. Tanzi. 2012. *Super Brain: Unleashing the Explosive Power of Your Mind to Maximize Health, Happiness, and Spiritual Well-Being.* London: Rider Books.

Desikachar, T.K.V. and R.H. Cravens. 2011. *Health, Healing and Beyond: Yoga and the Living Tradition of T. Krishnamacharya.* New York: North Point Press.

Gibran, Khalil. 2015. *The Broken Wings.* First Rate Publishers.

Hanh, Thich Nhat. 2009. *The Miracle of Mindfulness: The Classic Guide to Meditation by the World's Most Revered Master.* London: Rider Books.

Hanh, Thich Nhat. 2001. *Essential Writings.* New York: Orbis Books.

Iyengar, B.K.S. 2005. *Light on Life: The Yoga Journey to Wholesomeness, Inner Peace, and Ultimate Freedom.* USA: Rodale Inc.

Iyengar, B.K.S. 1993. *Light on the Yoga Sutras of Patanjali.* London: Thorsons.

Kaimal, Manoj. 2008. *Making Patanjali Palatable.* Manoj Kaimal.

Krishnamacharya, Tirumalai. 2016. *Yoga Makaranda: The Nectar of Yoga.* Chennai: Krishnamacharya Healing and Yoga Foundation.

Krishnamurti, Jiddu. 2003. *Krishnamurti on Education.* Chennai: Krishnamurti Foundation India.

'Manasa Yoga' *Teacher Training Notes.*

Mandela, Nelson. 1994. *Long Walk to Freedom.* Johannesburg, South Africa: Macdonald Purcell.

Paramahansa Yogananda. 2011. *God Talks With Arjuna: The Bhagavad Gita.* Kolkata: Yagoda Satsanga Society of India.

Sharma, Robin. 2009. *Who Will Cry When You Die?* Mumbai: Jaico Publishing House.

Swami Satchidananda. 1977. *Beyond Words.* Toronto: Holt, Rinehart & Winston of Canada Limited.

Swami Satchidananda, trans. 2004. *The Yoga Sutras of Patanjali.* USA: Integral Yoga Publications.

Tolle, Eckhart. 1999. *The Power of Now: A Guide to Spiritual Enlightenment.* Vancouver, Canada: Namaste Publishing and Novato, California: New World Library.

Weiss, Brian. 2000. *Only Love is Real: A Story of Soulmates Reunited.* New York: Warner Books, Inc.

Williamson, Marianne. 2006. *Everyday Grace: Having Hope, Finding Forgiveness and Making Miracles.* New York: Bantam Books.

Articles

Borchard, Therese J., 2010. The Old Man and His Horse. World of Psychology (blog), PsychCentral, https://psychcentral.com/blog/the-old-man-and-his-horse/

Chopra, Deepak. '5 Ways Meditation Can Make You Happier and More Successful at Work.' LinkedIn, July 19, 2013, https://www.linkedin.com/pulse/20130718224205-75054000-5-ways-meditation-can-make-you-happier/

DeWall, C. Nathan, Geoff Macdonald, Gregory D. Webster, Carrie L.

Masten, Roy F. Baumeister, Caitlin Powell, David Combs, David R. Schurtz, Tyler F. Stillman, Dianne M. Tice, and Naomi I. Eisenberger. 2010. Acetaminophen reduces social pain: behavioural and neural evidence. *Psychological Science* 21, issue 7: 931–37.

Hölzel, Britta K., James Carmody, Mark Vangel, Christina Congleton, Sita M. Yerramsetti, Tim Gard, and Sara W. Lazar. 2011. Mindfulness practice leads to increase in regional gray matter density. *Psychiatry Research* 191, issue 1:36–43.

Lazar, Sara W., Catherine E. Kerr, Rachel H. Wasserman, Jeremy R. Gray, Douglas N. Greve, Michael T. Treadway, Metta McGarvey, Brian T. Quinn, Jeffery A. Dusek, Herbert Benson, Scott L. Rauch, Christopher I. Moore, and Bruce Fischl. 2005. Meditation experience is associated with increased cortical thickness. *NeuroReport* 16, issue 17: 1893–97.

Luders, Eileen, Florian Kurth, Emeran A. Mayer, Arthur W. Toga, Katherine L. Narr, and Christian Gaser. 2012. The Unique Brain Anatomy of Meditation Practitioners: Alterations in Cortical Gyrification. *Frontiers in Human Neuroscience* 6, issue 34 (February 29), https://www.ncbi.nlm.nih.gov/pmc/articles/PMC3289949/

Luders, Eileen, Owen R. Phillips, Kristi Clark, Florian Kurth, Arthur W. Toga, and Katherine L. Narr. 2012. Bridging the hemispheres in meditation: thicker callosal regions and enhanced fractional anisotropy (FA) in long-term practitioners. *NeuroImage* 61, issue 1: 181–87.

Ruiz, Fernando Pagés. 2011. Krishnamacharya's Legacy. *Yoga Journal*, May/June issue.

Woollett, Katherine and Eleanor A. Maguire. 2011. Acquiring 'the Knowledge' of London's Layout Drives Structural Brain Changes. *Current Biology* 21, issue 24: 2109–14.